LIFE shifts

WOMEN'S STORIES OF SURRENDERING TO AND RISING ABOVE LIFE'S CHALLENGES

LINDA JOY

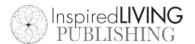

Inspired LIVING PUBLISHING

A Sacred Gift
to Support You on Your Self-Discovery Journey

Discover the power of energy-infused affirmations to elevate your mindset and create your intentional life.

Mindset Elevation *Intentional Life* Screensaver Set

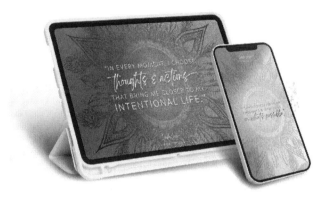

Your Mindset Elevation Affirmation Screensaver Set includes:

~5 energy-infused affirmation screensavers for your desktop or laptop

~5 energy-infused affirmation screensavers for your phone.

~Invitation to the Inspiration Lounge™ Facebook community

~VIP notice on future complimentary 5-day Mindset Elevation Soul Camps™

**It's time to say yes to igniting your inner mojo
and to living an intentional life!**

**Download your complimentary gift at:
www.MindsetElevationGiftSet.com**

i

ISBN: 978-1-7327425-8-1
ebook ISBN: 978-1-7327425-9-8
Library of Congress Control Number: Applied for

Published by Inspired Living Publishing, LLC.
P.O. Box 1149, Lakeville, MA 02347

Cover and interior design: Lisa Hromada (www.spiritledgraphicdesign.com)
Interior layout: Patricia Creedon (www.patcreedondesigns.com)
Managing Editor: Deborah Kevin, MA (www.deborahkevin.com)
Associate Editor: Adam Karofsky (www.askwrites.com)
Linda Joy photo credit: Ali Rosa Photography (www.alirosaphotography.com)

Dedication

This book is dedicated to:

Every woman who has experienced a life shift, or Cosmic 2x4, that brought her to her knees. I see you.

Every woman who has risen from the ashes to consciously create her life from a place of truth, courage, trust, and inner power. I honor you.

Every woman who has had to find the courage to step beyond her perceived limitations and into the unknown to find her way. I witness you.

And, also to:

Niki, my daughter, who inspires me daily with her loving and compassionate heart and as the sacred role model for her own daughter, Makenna.

Makenna (aka "The Little Goddess"), my spirited, creative, love-filled eleven-year-old granddaughter: May you always embrace your magic and magnificence, my love, and never dull your sparkle.

Tyler, my grandson: May you remember your truth and magic and find the greatest peace and happiness in that truth.

Dana, the love of my life: Twenty-nine years in and you still rock my world and melt my heart.

To the authors of *Life Shifts* who courageously said "yes" to diving deep and sharing their souls onto these pages to inspire every woman who reads their words.

The extraordinary team of talented individuals with whom I have been honored, blessed, and humbled to work with to bring this project to life: Deborah Kevin, chief editor on this sacred project, who brings the essence of each story to light and Adam Karofsky, associate editor for holding loving space for their stories to be told.

Lisa Hromada for the stunning cover and interior design, Patricia Creedon for the interior content layout, and Kim Turcotte, my Goddess of Operations and soul sister, who, for close to fifteen years, organizes and brings my visions to life.

And finally, to:

You, the reader—the deserving recipient of the love, light, and truth in these pages. May the words, vulnerability, and life wisdom that these women share empower you to see your value, hear your truth, and to follow the whispers of your soul.

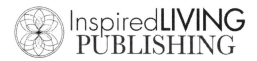
InspiredLIVING PUBLISHING

Also by Inspired Living Publishing

Inspired Living Publishing's bestselling titles include:

The Art of Self-Nurturing: A Field Guide to Living with More Peace, Joy & Meaning by Kelley Grimes, MSW

Broken Open: Embracing Heartache and Betrayal as Gateways to Unconditional Love by Mal Duane

Soul-Hearted Living: A Year of Sacred Reflections & Affirmations for Women by Dr. Debra Reble

Everything Is Going to Be Okay!: From the Projects to Harvard to Freedom by Dr. Catherine Hayes, CPCC

Being Love: How Loving Yourself Creates Ripples of Transformation in Your Relationship and the World by Dr. Debra Reble

Awakening to Life: Your Sacred Guide to Consciously Creating a Life of Purpose, Magic, and Miracles by Patricia Young

The Art of Inspiration: An Editor's Guide to Writing Powerful, Effective Inspirational & Personal Development Books, by Bryna Haynes

As well as these bestselling titles in our sacred anthology division:

Reclaiming Your Midlife Mojo: Women's Stories of Self-Discovery & Transformation

Life Reimagined! Women's Stories of Hope, Resilience & Transformation

SHINE! Stories to Inspire You to Dream Big, Fear Less & Blaze Your Own Trail

Courageous Hearts: Soul-Nourishing Stories to Inspire You to Embrace Your Fears and Follow Your Dreams

Midlife Transformation: Redefining Life, Love, Health and Success

Inspiration for a Woman's Soul: Opening to Gratitude & Grace

Inspiration for a Woman's Soul: Cultivating Joy

Inspiration for a Woman's Soul: Choosing Happiness

Embracing Your Authentic Self: Women's Stories of Self-Discovery & Transformation

A Juicy, Joyful Life: Inspiration from Women Who Have Found the Sweetness in Every Day

Unleash Your Inner Magnificence (ebook only)

The Wisdom of Midlife Women 2 (ebook only)

You can find most of the titles at major online retailers and bookstores by request.

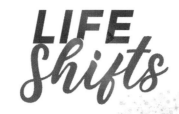

"The potent and vulnerable stories in *Life Shifts* will empower you to believe that, like the authors, within you lies the power, strength, and resilience to rise above life's curveballs. Curl up in your favorite chair with this transformational book and allow their stories to open your heart to what's possible."

AMY LEIGH MERCREE

Medical intuitive and bestselling author of eighteen books, including *The Healing Home, Aura Alchemy,* and the card deck *Blissful Baths: 40 Rituals for Self-Care and Relaxation*

"*Life Shifts* is a truly inspiring book of women's stories that will remind you that, above all else, always listen to and honor the wisdom of your intuition. That awareness does not only enter our consciousness but speaks loudly through our bodies. Listen, follow, and trust that guidance from within, always."

EMILY A. FRANCIS

Author and wellness advocate

"Know what I love? Women sharing from their hearts to uplift other women. As Lisa Hromada writes in her lovely account of learning to dance with the Universe, 'Just maybe I am here to create something powerful.' If you have picked up this book, just maybe you are, too."

LISA MCCOURT
Author of *Free Your Joy* and founder of Joy School

"Reading this empowered collection of heart-centered *Life Shifts* reignites that ineffable, shared spark of possibility, fueled by a lifetime of sometimes-silent longing for the lived experience filled with hope, connection, and healing. Each story shares the same thread of inspiration: It is possible to begin living your most aligned life at any moment."

NANCI REED
Sacred embodiment coach and author

"Another stunning collection of inspiring stories from courageous 'guided by spirit' women writers. Linda Joy has done it again— curating in a conscious and highly intentional way, compiling a book you'll want on your bedside for those moments when you most need to receive confirmation that you aren't crazy— you are connected!"

ANJEL B. HARTWELL
The Wealthy Life Mentor

"As your soul yearns for growth and evolution, the radiant intelligence of love extends a tender invitation, beckoning you to embrace a deeper truth about your essence. A powerful collection of relatable stories, *Life Shifts* is your companion on the path of self-discovery towards living your authentic, empowered, true nature."

JEANINE THOMPSON

Former Fortune 50 executive, transformational coach, speaker,
and award-winning author of *911 From Your Soul*

"In her powerful new anthology, *Life Shifts*, Linda Joy has once again curated a collection of women's stories of courage, resilience, and transformation. These vulnerable yet empowering stories show us how to embrace life's challenges and use them to create soul-inspired life shifts. Every story empowers you to be the artist of your own life by providing inspiration, real life examples, and spiritual lessons to support you on your soul's journey. *Life Shifts* reminds you, that you alone have the power within you to co-create a purposeful, happy, and joy-filled life."

DR. DEBRA L. REBLE

Intuitive psychologist, transformational life coach, and
bestselling author

"Abundant wisdom you can soak up and utilize in your own life. The authors' stories in *Life Shifts* draw you right in. The women share right from their souls and capture your heart. So raw, honest, and authentic—as the reader, you find so many feelings and experiences you relate to. Just beautiful."

DR. COLLEEN GEORGES

Coach, author, and TEDx speaker

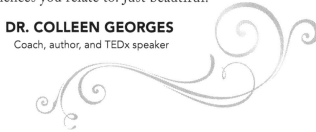

"As a fifty-eight-year-old woman, I can no longer keep track of the many potent life shifts I have experienced. The stories in this book reminded me of the potent transformation that happens at pivotal moments and that there is always light and growth on the other side of challenge. I particularly liked the story, "Learning to Dance with the Universe," a powerful reminder to believe in ourselves and trust the divine calling we are given. Another fabulous compilation book by Linda Joy full of inspirational stories and meaningful lessons for navigating life's shifts."

MINETTE RIORDAN, PhD
Midlife transformation coach, artist, and author

"*Life Shifts* happen when we listen to our inner wisdom, our intuition, our hearts' whisper. The stories in this book are testimony that illustrate what can happen and how we can live the life we are meant to have when we go within."

APRIL GOFF BROWN
Human Design life coach

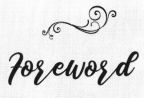

Foreword

BY KRISTI LING SPENCER

*S*everal years ago, I found myself navigating a tidal wave of grief and heartbreak after the unraveling of my decade-long marriage. It was crushing and relentless. One especially tough morning, I had to absolutely force myself to slither out of bed and scoop myself up off of the floor to face the day. I knew I needed nutrition to keep my immune system afloat, and a fresh green juice was about the only thing that sounded doable to me in the moment.

I put on some frumpy sweats, tied up my chaotic hair, and made my way to the Organic Café down the street. As I reached the counter, I asked the server in what was likely the bluest-sounding voice she'd ever heard, "Do you have any juices with kale, spinach, and lemon?"

She perkily replied back, "We sure do! It's called the Learn to Let Go!"

The irony stopped my spinning brain in its tracks. A spontaneous laugh escaped my mouth and she laughed along with me. "Okay, good name!" I answered. I'd actually forgotten what it felt like to laugh, and it was a welcome reminder. I took my drink and as I walked away, I whispered, "Okay, got it. Thanks for the hint.

I'll keep going."

Sometimes the support we need to lift us up at just the right time comes from decidedly unexpected places, if we're open. By picking up *Life Shifts,* you've opened yourself to fresh insights, beautiful connection, and even powerful support that might come from just one story or even a single sentence.

Life can have a such distinctive way of presenting us with colossal challenges and curveballs when we're least expecting them. They're the things that can turn an ordinary day, week, or even year into the perfect storm. Sometimes they're things we've known were on the way, but are never fully prepared for when they happen. And, sometimes they're completely unexpected events that blindside us on a quiet Wednesday.

For women, these challenges can be even more multifaceted and layered, as we navigate the intricacies of societal expectations, gender biases, and our own personal dreams and aspirations.

The beautiful truth is that within every challenge—even the ones we wish we'd never experienced—are opportunities for incredible growth, healing, and transformation.

In this powerful book imagined by the amazing Linda Joy, we embark on a journey—an exploration of the depths of our collective strength and the invincible spirit of women who have risen above life's unexpected challenges.

Throughout these pages, you will encounter personal stories of extraordinary women who have confronted diverse challenges—broken hearts, shattered dreams, major setbacks, health crises, and personal loss. Their narratives are not just tales of incredible resilience and triumph, but inspiring accounts of lessons and personal growth. These women have demonstrated that it's possible to not only get through life's hardships, but to also emerge stronger, wiser, and more empowered than before.

As you delve into their stories, you will discover universal themes that resonate deeply: resilience, courage, perseverance, intuition, and the unwavering belief that we possess the strength to overcome any obstacle. Through their journeys, you will find solace, inspiration, and practical wisdom you can apply to your own life.

This book is a true celebration of the unconquerable essence of women.

Let these stories be a guiding light on your own path. Let them remind you that you're stronger than you realize, and you're never alone. It's my sincerest hope that as you read these accounts, you will find comfort, inspiration, and a renewed sense of belief in your own ability to rise above any adversity that comes your way. Enjoy the beautiful gifts you're about to receive.

With love, support, and light,

Kristi Ling Spencer
Bestselling Author of *Operation Happiness*,
Keynote Speaker, Host of *The Joy School Podcast*
@kristilingspencer | kristilingspencer.com

Table of Contents

Introduction

$\mathcal{S}$itting in my car on a warm spring day in 1991, I experienced a transformational life shift, or Cosmic 2x4, and discovered the healing power of choice.

I've often said that my life, and my soul's work, began that day as I sobbed against my steering wheel on the side of a tree-lined road. As I cried out to the Divine for help, I was given an epiphany. One that rocked my inner world and began my healing journey. I could choose to continue as I was—a self-sabotaging welfare mom of a six-year-old, carrying wounds from my traumatic past, a woman without direction or hope for her own future—or I could choose something different. The choice was mine to make.

My life shift moment—one of many—had arrived.

The empowering, sacred truth that was revealed that day— I have a *choice* about how I experience my life—filled my heart with hope and forever changed the trajectory of my life. Today, it continues to fuel my work as a mindset elevation coach, publisher of *Aspire Magazine*, storytelling guide, bestselling publisher at Inspired Living Publishing, and the host of numerous other inspirational media brands—all dedicated to publishing content that reminds women of the truth of who they are, encourages them to believe in possibility and inspires them to become the author of their own story.

Little did I know that on that spring day over thirty-two years ago, I'd be inspired and led to the magical and empowering work with women that I'm blessed to do today. Looking back, I can see that my darkest day led me to my soul's light and the mission-driven work I am passionate about.

Out of the darkness, I found MY light.

Over the last seventeen years since founding *Aspire Magazine*, I've met and heard from thousands of empowered women who have created authentic, joyful, inspiring lives for themselves and their families. While these women have each traveled their own unique paths and overcome their own pain, obstacles, and perceived failures, their stories still seem to have a common thread. At some point in her life, each woman experienced her "life shift moment" and then made a pivotal choice of some kind, a conscious decision that changed her life and her role within it.

As I shared in the introduction to ILP's bestselling anthology, *Courageous Hearts:*

At some point, we are all called to make choices—about our careers, relationships, health, and how we appear in the world. These choices determine how we create our personal realities. However, it is often not until we are at our most vulnerable, our most fragile, that we can hear the soft but inevitable calling of our hearts. What we choose in those moments has the power to keep us stuck in a life that no longer fits who we are—or ignites our authentic selves and opens the way to a life beyond what we ever imagined.

My life shift moment catapulted me into my power. I chose, moment by moment, to release the story of self-sabotage, victimhood, and fear and to rewrite a new story for myself of courage, resilience, inner strength, and grace. It's a journey that continues today.

Beautiful soul, even in the midst of the darkest night, when everything is falling apart, our power to choose our reactions and our peace is still available. Sometimes, it's not until we hit rock bottom that we see the choice before us—but sometimes, all it takes is a gentle reminder that we are powerful, lovable, and worthy enough to create our lives and ourselves in the image of the Divine and according to our souls' plans.

The stories in this sacred compilation are the soul-inspiring truths of women who have been there, done that, and come out the other side more vital than ever. They share their transformational stories of breaking through the barriers imposed upon themselves so that they can choose love and self-empowerment over fear and constriction. They are stories of loss, healing, love, and surrender. They are stories from women, just like you, who found the strength to follow their heart's whispers, and whose lives and dreams blossomed as a result.

I hope you will see some part of yourself in their stories and understand that the empowered choices these ladies have made are yours to make. May their stories remind you of your strength, courage, resilience, and inner strength so that when life throws you a curve ball, you can hold your head up high, look in the mirror and say, "I've got this."

Joy, healing, happiness, love, and intentional living are yours for the taking.

All you have to do is choose!

Live an Intentional Life!
Linda Joy
Mindset Elevation Coach
Storytelling Guide and Bestselling Publisher
www.Linda-Joy.com

CHAPTER ONE
Shifting Mindset

A Costly Mistake: Ignoring My Inner Wisdom

KAREN SHIER

*I*t was 2008. Markets crashed. The economy plummeted. The company where I'd served for two years as a director of Human Resources struggled to weather the economic storm. Many of its nationwide branch offices closed, resulting in dozens of employees being laid off.

A colleague privately shared with me that he had put his résumé out there … just in case. Pay cuts were shared by all employees, with even larger cuts handed to the management team. My ex-husband stopped paying child support. My income dwindled, yet I still had a mortgage, automobile, and student loans to pay monthly.

My blonde-haired, green-eyed daughter, having just been diagnosed with ADHD, struggled both with focus and bullies at school. I remained stalwart in my endeavors to keep her safe, secure, and forward-focused.

Amid this maelstrom came the crushing blow.

In my desire to create a better retirement future than I had witnessed growing up, I, at the age of twenty-one, made biweekly deposits into my company's 401(k) retirement plan. I worked in the banking industry and understood that saving for my future was the right thing to do, even on my meager salary.

When I moved to the HR director role, I believed I needed to diversify my retirement funds. Perhaps I mistrusted my new company on some level, or maybe I absorbed unverified or misguided information from others.

No matter what my reasons, instead of rolling over my existing 401(k) into my new company's plan, I moved my entire balance into a self-directed IRA at an investment company that was a "can't-go-wrong-sure-thing" at the advice of a close and trusted friend.

I ignored my shouting gut feeling, suppressing the inner wisdom that communicated to me through my emotional body. "Don't do it," my gut screamed while my mind rationalized my decision.

Instead, I allowed my inner critic to take control and listened to my thoughts like "put your money here because you don't know what else to do" and "you don't have the smarts or the time to invest these funds on your own" and other insidious whisperings my ego used in its attempt to keep me safely in my comfort zone. I also got caught up in the exciting possibility of this "sure thing."

Thoughts like these whirled around in my head:

- When the "guaranteed" returns started flowing, I'd have a wonderful retirement;

- I wouldn't have to work into my eighties like my grandmother had;

- I'd experience financial freedom, not the scrimping and scraping I'd grown up with; and

- How joyfully secure I'd feel once the financial windfall showered down.

Those difficult internal arguments between my head and my gut continued until my head accepted my gut's unconditional surrender. I moved all my retirement savings, all the while ignoring the instinct that something didn't feel right.

After investing my entire retirement balance into the "sure thing" IRA, all seemed well for about a year. I received monthly statements showing my balance climbing nicely. I never before imagined seeing that much money in my own account. I felt accomplished and smart for having made this move.

And then, in 2009, my friend confided change was coming and suggested I might want to move my funds into something else.

Crap! I was ineligible to roll my money into my company's 401(k) plan because of the laws surrounding the timing of moving retirement funds. I didn't have time to research new options with the hours I worked and responsibilities I had. I didn't have the smarts to invest on my own. I couldn't afford an adviser. I didn't know where to turn.

At least those are the things I told myself. So, I remained paralyzed until that pit in my gut forced me to take action. I reached out to the investment company to withdraw my funds and requested my full $110,000 balance. They said they could only give me $30,000. After a few weeks, they sent me a check for $15,000, promising the rest would come soon. That check bounced. Then they sent me another $10,000, and—no surprise—that check also bounced.

The investment company stopped answering my emails and phone calls. My online account access no longer worked. I grew increasingly panicked, and that pit in my stomach seemed to bore a hole right through me. Immense fear and anxiety took over. Something was definitely wrong.

My banker advised me that he suspected something fraudulent was happening and encouraged me to contact the FBI. My worst fears came true. Was I going to have to retain an expensive attorney? I certainly wasn't in any position to be able to afford that.

Fortunately, I had taken copious notes on my dealings with the investment company. The FBI investigator called me back and told me that they were involved in a joint criminal investigation with the SEC and IRS. My name was added to the growing list of victims in what appeared to be a huge criminal fraud case.

I'm a victim? Ouch!

The agent shared that the FBI had frozen the assets of the owners but at the time estimated these assets totaled only 1 percent of what they believed these people had hidden all over the world in a Ponzi scheme arrangement. All of the monthly account statements I saw were bogus. My heart sank.

At one point in the investigation, the agent told me he figured that my life savings were probably spent within three days. Talk about disheartening. I felt so angry, stupid, powerless, and guilty at my bad financial decision. *How could I have let this happen?* I felt so alone.

In 2011, I testified in federal court as a credible witness. This group of scammers had gained the trust of hundreds of people, gladly took our money, and squandered away our life savings in a matter of months.

As I looked around the depressingly dark and packed courtroom, I realized I was likely the youngest of over 700 people who had been defrauded. Many had already retired and had only social security to fall back on. Some had passed away, never knowing the outcome of this horrific event on our lives.

Although I crumbled inside, unsure how I would recover from the financial blow, the FBI agents commended me on my calm professionalism and even asked me if I would be willing to coach other victims through the experience. Of course, I'd be happy to help if I could.

I realized that although this was probably one of the more traumatic events that had happened to me, I was only forty-four years old. I still had some time to save again, to regain some of what I had lost. And perhaps, like my grandmother, I may work well past the age I had hoped to, but I could, and I would if I had to.

Many of the other victims didn't have that option; the trajectory of their lives had changed forever.

Unfortunately, I didn't know the extent of the physical toll those chronic financial stresses took on my mind, body, and soul. That wouldn't show up fully until years later.

Today, I'm more than okay. I have processed my anger, forgiven myself, and put it behind me. I continue to save and have the support of my wonderful husband. Together, we are building a secure retirement future.

I no longer pontificate on how much money I could have had in my retirement account. It no longer matters because I have since learned that money is just energy, and it will flow again as I joyfully expect it to. I know in my heart we will be just fine.

The beautiful lesson for me to this day remains: soothe my inner critic first and only listen to my heart's whisperings, as these will always point me in the right direction.

Reflection:

What have you experienced in your life that became a pivotal wake-up call for you?

Can you remember a time when you didn't follow your intuition and things didn't go so well for you? Looking back, what might you have done differently?

Can you remember a time that you did follow your intuition and things went really well for you? How did that make you feel?

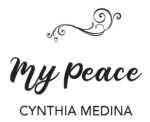

My Peace

CYNTHIA MEDINA

*I*t was a gorgeous spring morning, and I was sitting out on my back porch listening to the birds. With a cup of coffee in my hand, I sat there and felt a peace wash over me. A peace that I had never encountered before in this lifetime. A feeling that was so foreign yet, in a way, so familiar. It felt like home.

I haven't had an easy journey in this life. From my entrance into this world until my late forties, I experienced numerous challenges. Some were basic human challenges that everyone faces, and others I never could have seen coming. Through these struggles, I attached to the core beliefs of "I am not good enough" and "The world isn't safe."

While these core beliefs made my journey incredibly difficult at times, I never let them completely hold me back. I knew deep inside of me that I had a purpose. I was driven by a deep passion to love and, along with the negative core beliefs, I held some pretty strong positive ones as well: "Love can heal" and "All we need is love!" These beliefs were my saving grace; they got me to where I am today.

I was always a natural-born leader. You see, I had a dream. I saw the suffering of others and wanted to create something incredible to comfort the ones that were losing hope, feeling betrayed by the medical system and, quite frankly, their own bodies. I set out on a journey to start an integrative wellness center in my mid-twenties with no model to follow. I was on my own journey to get well at the same time. My body had, in many ways, betrayed me, and I was driven to find answers to help myself and help others.

Embarking on this journey while raising a family began to reveal my deeply held wounds, and I was on a search for answers. As an empath, there were times I was taking on the pain of others as well as my own, and I had to learn how to navigate the energies within and around me. My nervous system was my gauge. For many years I thought my body was against me, but I later realized my body held the secrets to my healing and, ultimately, the peace I would one day begin to feel.

There were many shifts along the way as I tested my world, the concept of "love," and what it means. I became a lover of psychology. Why is it so hard for people to feel safe in this world and just love one another? This was the burning question I needed the answer to. As you can imagine, when you ask a question like this, the Universe will respond with the lessons to lead to the answers—many will confuse you and many will delight you, and even some will torment you.

Today as I look back upon my life, I can see that I was fully supported and protected by the Universe. Were there some horrifying life-altering experiences along the way? Of course, there were, and they shook me to my core. But they were answering my questions as well in their own way. You see, pain, love, fear, and trust can all exist simultaneously.

As a deeply intuitive being, I feel everything to the extreme and try to understand what it all means. How do we operate as a being with a mind, body, and soul? How do we fluctuate from our physical self to our spiritual self? How do our brains and our minds show up in their unique ways? And how do our bodies measure our own spiritual self-frequency? I look at the communication that exists between all the aspects of who we are. I see how we self-regulate and create a flow between everything we do, think, feel, and believe. This energy flow is incredible, and when you're in tune, you feel it.

It was only when I began to love and value myself that I saw the world as a place of enlightenment. When I shifted to the position of being connected to the great source of all, I knew that I had permission to claim my mission here in this existence. I had to forge ahead without the permission or acceptance of others, and even without their understanding. I had to let go of everyone else's beliefs, ideals, and values for me.

Of course, when you have an awakening, you will often encounter many things that make you question if you are on the right path. Life will challenge you to see how strong you are in your faith and your belief in your purpose. I am no exception. After shifting away from the stories I had created, I encountered many blessings, yet I also faced the most horrifying experiences of my life. Only those of you reading this who have lost a child will truly understand. And, as a double whammy, I then lost my ability to walk for a season after a virus attacked my legs. At this point, I was cracked wide open, vulnerable. I didn't even really know who I was anymore.

As another layer of self-doubt and fear was peeled open, I had to face the fact that I did not have any control over what may come my way without warning and alter my life dramatically. This poked again at my core beliefs. You see, these events were sudden, shocking, and drove me to a deep understanding that I had to surrender to survive. The illusion that I had any control was ripped from me at every level. All I had control over was my ability to love and maintain my attitude and energy at a high level. I couldn't walk, I couldn't see the future of my condition, I couldn't do the things I needed to do for myself. All I could do was surrender and love.

I was faced with accepting my new self. The self that was no longer able to dance, wear heels and dress up and present to the world. The self that had to rely on people to assist me. The self that now lived with daily physical pain. The self that didn't really know where this child went. The self that couldn't be the mother I was or the wife I was. The self that had to surrender and hope that others had the kind of love for me that I had envisioned and dreamed for the world.

I was vulnerable, and yet I had to survive. I decided that I would recreate myself. I started a new business and worked from my bed until I could walk again. I was not going to be a victim, and if I wanted to heal, I had to take charge of my healing myself. I could no longer focus on what I couldn't do, but instead focused on what was possible and what I wanted to create.

The years weren't easy. I faced other challenges. But with each one I overcame, my faith, belief, and love for myself and others increased. I began to trust myself to get through whatever life would throw at me. I began to see this life as working for me, not against me. I began to see that I had the power to love even in the most gut-wrenching situations.

This brings me back to that spring day, sitting on my porch, listening to the birds sing, sipping my coffee, and feeling the greatest level of peace. Today I can walk. Gratitude floods my being every day. I surrender to the flow and the experience of this life. And as my life shifts, I will embrace each new experience with grace and ease giving thanks and knowing I am wrapped in the unconditional love of Source. I know myself and my mission, and it is my anchor. I am here to give love, receive love, and make a difference in the life of each person who crosses my path. I am the energy and embodiment of love, and nothing that happens in this life can take that away from me. This is my deepest peace.

Reflection:

Have you identified your core beliefs? How has knowing your values helped you navigate life?

How has a loss of a loved one shaped your lived experience?

How do you define love and how does your definition serve you?

Learning to Surf

SHA BLACKBURN

I grew up on a dirt road in a small town with a pond for my front yard and woods for the back. I boated, swam, fished, ice skated, and felt comfortable on the little freshwater pond where I lived. Even though we sailed, and powerboated as a family, I never had the desire to captain more than my kayak. Despite being descended from mariners, I never felt that part of my DNA.

In 2013, I was fortunate enough to go to Hawaii, and the only thing I really wanted to do was learn to surf. My friend Sherrie, a founding member of my coven who had passed away several years prior, had been an avid surfer. She and I learned how to ride motorcycles together and used to go out together as single ladies, with me often playing her wingwoman. Sherrie had an infectious love of life! I keep a small amount of her ashes on my ancestral shrine—one of the few who are blessed to have a place of honor there. I took her cremains with me to Hawaii. She always wanted to surf there, and I couldn't pass up the opportunity to share my adventure with her.

One of my best friends, Lisa, traveled with me to Hawaii. She had a time-share, and I only had to pay for airfare, as everything else was covered except whatever sightseeing we wanted to do.

Lisa and I decided that we were going to go take a surf lesson. Lisa had been hit by a car a few years before our trip and had lost the function of her left arm and hand.

We made our reservation and went down to a small beach in a little cove where the waves were pretty easygoing, so not a hot surf spot for avid surfers. It proved a perfect place to learn pretty safely. Although I grew up sailing and boating of all sorts, I wasn't a big fan of putting myself in the ocean on purpose because there are things that are definitely on the top of the food chain OVER ME that live in there. I have a healthy respect for the ocean and all her power to sweep one away if she deems it so.

Our instructor was a small, well-built surfer dude, who was a total riot teaching these two old ladies all the techniques of surfing. He marveled at the fact that Lisa was going to give surfing a try.

She said, "I'm only doing it to keep Sha out of trouble and to make sure she has the courage to do it."

When I make up my mind to tackle something, 99 percent of the time, I do it come hell or high water. Lisa and I have a complex relationship that I don't understand most of the time. Lisa can be protective of me, and when she couldn't take care of herself, I took care of her. So, I let her watch out for me, and I let her love me. She is more of a sister to me than a friend, if I am being honest.

The instructor showed us how to jump up to our feet from lying on our stomachs. I don't know who he thought was going to accomplish that, but certainly not forty-four-year-old me!

I said, "I can get on my knees that fast but will never get on my feet. And Lisa here certainly isn't going to be able to do that either. Can we surf on our knees?"

He said, "I believe in you."

I laughed again—he had mirrored back to me what I tell others—and I said, "I will be able to do it someday, but since I haven't been able to do that in the first forty-four years of my life, today probably IS NOT the day that I suddenly will."

He smiled at that and said, "Okay. If you think you can get to your knees, go for it, but don't think you can't get on your feet if you really want to."

I paddled out into the ocean while Lisa got towed out. We turned ourselves around and watched the waves over our shoulders while we straddled our boards. I felt such a rush of energy—joy, peace, anticipation, harmony—it took my breath away.

Our instructor said, "Okay! See it, here it comes."

I laid down and started paddling.

The instructor was behind me and yelled, "PADDLE HARD NOW!" before giving me a shove.

I paddled like my hands were on fire; the wave came under me, I got to my knees and felt myself fly. There are few times in my life when I have had such a freedom of body and soul. I squealed and sang and shouted and smiled ... and couldn't wait to get out and do it again.

When Lisa came in, I cheered her on as if I was on the board with her—I felt all the same amazing sensations. WOW! When Lisa was about to give up, I towed her back out behind me so we could surf again. I towed her out twice, and I surfed about half a dozen waves myself. I could have stayed and surfed until the sun set, and it still wouldn't have been enough for me. I found my familial connection to the sea and felt myself deeply grounded by this alignment to the primordial waters of life. I don't think I ever knew true freedom until that moment when the first wave lifted me up and taught me to fly.

I dreamed of surfing. I dreamed of Hawaii. I can put myself there again and again in my mind and feel those same feelings. So, that year for my birthday, when my boyfriend asked me what I wanted, I said, "A surfboard," not thinking he would actually buy one for me ... but he did! And I have surfed at least once a year since I got the board, except that first year when I spent the summer practicing my paddling, straddling, falling off, unleash-

23

ing, and really studied about the waves and the tides so I would be strong and ready when I finally got out there.

I still have never gotten on my feet, though a few people have tried to teach and encourage me. I don't know why that skill eludes me—probably because it's hard since I am not in shape to do it, but someday I will. Even when I fell off and the board clunked me three times pretty hard on the head and I thought to myself, "Shit, this is how people drown," I never have a fear of getting back out there. I don't think about the sharks and jellyfish and all the other sea creatures who could hurt me; I just think about the connection I feel, the energy that courses through me when I am riding the waves on my board, the freedom that runs through my whole self.

I bought prescription swim goggles so that it will be a bit easier for me to get out on the water; I won't have the limitation of my poor sight. Fingers crossed; I'll continue to get out there at least once a summer because it recharges me like lightning striking the earth. It reminds me that I am totally FREE, and that I am one part of a larger whole that I can find harmony and balance within.

Reflection:

What's something you've always wanted to try or do but haven't? What's stopping you?

Think of a time when you tried something new, but it didn't work the first time. What messages did you give yourself about your value in that experience? How might you reframe it today?

How does perfectionism stop you from trying new things?

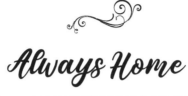

Always Home

SHARON KATHRYN D'AGOSTINO

*A*rmed soldiers were on both sides of the road from the airport to the capital city. It was not the welcome I had expected. I had long wanted to visit this country whose rich history and traditions fascinated me, and I was excited about the possibilities of what the upcoming days might hold.

The hotel where I would be staying sent someone to pick me up. Kilometer after kilometer, we passed soldiers evenly spaced, holding their weapons across their chests. I wondered why they were there and if I should be concerned. I had seen armed guards in other countries, including my own, but never as many as that road. I felt frightened.

I asked the taxi driver, "Is this a usual occurrence?"

He said it was not.

Relieved, I asked, "Have you seen this before?"

He looked into the rearview mirror, smiled, and asked me about my flight, clearly indicating that we would not discuss the soldiers and the guns. What, I thought, could be more important than the reason these soldiers were guarding the road? Instead, we talked about unimportant things and acted as though there was nothing unusual about riding past all of these soldiers and the weapons they held. Nothing had happened to me, so I wasn't allowing the presence of soldiers to diminish my enthusiasm for this city or this country. At least, I didn't think so.

Checking into the hotel was easy. As I handed my passport to the hotel manager, I asked him about the soldiers.

The manager smiled and replied, "Perhaps a foreign dignitary or a delegation of dignitaries is arriving today."

I had time to freshen up before joining colleagues, a few who lived locally and others from neighboring countries. After several hours of meetings, we enjoyed a late dinner, and our local colleagues shared mesmerizing stories about their culture, customs, and family traditions. No one could explain the presence of so many soldiers.

Early the following day, four of us traveled to meet colleagues working several hours away. When we arrived, a kind woman welcomed us and said, "You should know that a bomb exploded in a tourist area of the capital city today." She continued speaking, but I did not hear another word. I immediately thought of my parents. They always worried when I traveled out of our home country. I quickly calculated the time difference and decided nothing would frighten my parents more than being awakened by a phone call in the middle of the night.

I sat through meetings, watching the time. When it would have been 7:00 a.m. at home, I called.

My dad answered immediately, and in his "Hello," I could hear his fear. I felt his fear.

"Hi, Dad. You may hear about an explosion that happened in the capital city today. I was nowhere near it. I was not even in the city when it happened. Please don't worry. I am safe."

"We heard about it last night," he said, his voice shaking. "Your mother and I didn't sleep all night."

I felt terrible. "I'm fine, Dad, and safe. I am so sorry that you and Mom were worried. You know that you can always call my cell phone when I am traveling." Our conversation continued, and then I talked with my mom. "This is a beautiful city in a beautiful country," I told her. "Everything is fine, and I am completely safe." As I spoke these words, I felt the truth of them. I was not just trying to keep my parents from worrying. I knew that there was nothing to fear. Nothing.

When the call ended, I sobbed. A colleague tried to console me, but I was distraught. I felt responsible for my parents' worry, responsible that I had caused them a sleepless night. I was upset that I hadn't called them earlier, even though it had been in the middle of the night. I realize now that these regrets were not helpful to me or them, but I acknowledge that I had them.

The following day, my colleagues left for the airport several hours before me, and I continued to work before heading to the lobby to return my room key. I had been advised not to call a taxi, and the hotel had arranged for a trusted driver to take me to the airport. The driver was scheduled to arrive within ten minutes.

Few people were in the lobby. I noticed a bouquet of colorful flowers and sat down beside them in a chair against the back wall. I was anxious to leave, and every one of the ten minutes passed slowly, and then another ten minutes, and then another fifteen. Before I knew it, it was thirty-five minutes later. I went to the front desk to inquire about the delay.

"Oh, I am sure he will be here soon," the manager said.

Soon? I went back to my seat and waited impatiently. I became aware of saying something repeatedly in my mind, a silent mantra. "I want to go home. I want to go home. I want to go home." Where was that driver? I wanted to leave, and he still hadn't arrived. The inward chanting continued, "I want to go home. I want to go home. I want to go home."

Then, I heard a voice that was crystal clear. She spoke only four words, but every one of them was as resonant as a beautiful bell, "You are always home."

Reflexively, I turned my head to look behind me. Even as I did, I knew that no one was there; only a wall was behind me. No

29

one was near enough for me to hear their conversation. A stillness came over me, and my worries and fears evaporated. I felt relieved and grateful, as if I had been transported to a new reality. I heard none of the sounds that had been present in the lobby just moments before. I was enfolded in a deep peace and tranquility that I had never experienced.

The voice and her message changed me. I was totally calm, and I realized the truth of her words and their transformative power. I AM always home. It took some time for me to understand that, in that moment, my soul reminded me to be fully present in the now and to appreciate what was happening within and around me, not what should happen or could happen or had already happened. I understood that waiting in the lobby, I could have chosen to face the bouquet of fragrant flowers instead of staring at the hotel entrance expecting the driver to appear. The choice had been mine.

Over the following days and weeks, other interpretations of the words blossomed in my awareness. "You are always home" took on new meanings and guided me into the next stage of my spiritual journey. I had always been a driven individual with many responsibilities and expectations for myself. While the message was about always being home, it reminded me of other truths in my life. I interpreted it to also mean that I did not need to be someplace where I was not. I did not need to search for something that was beyond my grasp. It was all here. I also realized that I was not responsible for other people's decision to worry, not even my beloved parents.

The most important lesson was that I had, and always have, the power to decide what to feel and where to focus my attention. I can always be grateful to be exactly where I am and exactly who I am, and not who others expect me to be. I am always home.

Reflection:

Have you ever visited someplace new and felt unsafe? How did you respond and react?

What is your definition of "home?" Has this view changed over time? If so, how?

When someone's perception of you conflicts with your self-perception, what tools do you use to stay true to yourself?

It's Never Too Late

CINDY WINSEL

I was twenty-seven years old and excited about a new adventure. I had been teaching for a few years in the US when I decided to volunteer to teach abroad. Officially, I would be collaborating with teachers in a developing country, helping them work with students with learning disabilities. But really, I was there to help in any way I could. The small village in Costa Rica I was assigned to had very few supplies for teachers and their students, so I knew I'd have my work cut out for me.

Although I was living in a house owned by a man from the United States, it was nothing like what I was used to. In the village, all the houses were open, meaning there were no windows. On any given day I would have cockroaches, frogs, chickens, and other assorted animals living with me.

The owner of my new home was close with the family who lived next door, even paying for one of their children to go to the United States to study. He had completed his education and was now back living with his family. This man was around my age, and we soon became friends. He helped me with my Spanish, and I helped him with his English. When I started teaching English classes to the locals, he helped me promote them to the community.

Although the work I was doing was challenging, it was so rewarding. I made amazing connections with my fellow teachers and our students. Many of the local teachers sought me out as an expert, but I always collaborated with them as equals, ensuring we were working as a team to ensure student success. I always prided myself on my ability to build relationships back home, and this village was no different.

And then it all changed. One night, while I slept, this man, whom I thought of as a friend, came into my home and forced himself on me. I yelled, "NO!" and thought to myself, "How is this happening to me?" I let my mind and my body go somewhere else. I thought about home and the smell of bacon when my dad would cook breakfast. And then I lay still until the smell of his sweat left me.

When he left, I fled. I threw all my belongings into my duffel bag and got on the first bus I could find. In my panicked state, all I could think about was how this bus reminded me of a movie where the lead character rides a bus on a very rugged road in a foreign country, surrounded by mothers, crying babies, chickens, and goats. My bus out of there was exactly the same.

Once I made it to San José, I called my mom and dad and briefly told them what had happened. I don't think they really understood, but they heard the turmoil in my voice, and they said the words I needed to hear.

"Come home."

At twenty-seven, I left home, excited for a new adventure. I came home wounded physically, emotionally, spiritually, and mentally. I felt like a failure.

I pushed being raped down inside me and lied to myself that I had dealt with it. I compartmentalized my life between professional and personal and built an extraordinarily successful thirty-five-year teaching career. I knew my stuff and was good at what I did. I excelled.

I knew I wanted to be a teacher from a very early age. Nothing was going to stop me from realizing this goal. Once I started teaching, I put all my energy into being successful with my students. I focused on my relationships with colleagues, students, and parents. I felt needed, and I received positive feedback on my work. I loved planning out my lessons, collaborating with my colleagues, and working with students and their parents. Perhaps it was the structure of this profession that was comforting. As a teacher, I always felt wanted and because of this, I put every ounce of energy into my profession. My relationships at school were more important than my other relationships. I was loved and respected and didn't get that anywhere else. I flourished and lived every aspect of my life for student success.

In my personal life, however, I struggled. I struggled with my relationships with men. I fell into romantic relationships quickly, each time thinking I had found "the one."

My first husband was abusive, and my second husband was an addict. I had such low self-esteem that any man that came along I was ready to go full in with a relationship, whether it was healthy or not.

I intuitively knew that my second marriage was not going to last; however, I didn't have the energy to deal with it. My marriage was unhealthy, and my alcohol use was increasing, so I continued to do what I had always done: push my feelings down and numb them with alcohol.

It took a while before the personal and professional parts of my life came together, but eventually, it happened. The trauma of the rape, my second marriage ending, and my alcohol dependence created the perfect storm to be shaken awake. I chose to step into my healing process and realized I needed help and balance in my life.

To kickstart my healing, I needed to start finding out who I really was and find out how to love myself. I've done several different forms of therapy, and they have all helped, but along my journey, I had one therapist that got right to the point.

She sat me down and said, "You have not dealt with your rape."

35

I could have run away, but I decided to lean in and do the work this time. My entire world was falling apart, and deep down I knew I would have to deal with all the parts of me to become healthy. It took several months of one-on-one therapy for me to do the intense work that was required for me to release the pain, shame, and low self-worth. It took time for me to embrace all the wonderful parts of myself. I was beginning to feel whole.

The next piece of my healing process was to look at my alcohol use. Using alcohol was no longer aligned with my new journey. To continue to close all the wounds and to finally find freedom, comfort, and peace, I surrendered to my Higher Power to show me the way. That way was through a twelve-step program. I am now eight years sober!

The rape impacted my life in more ways than I realized. It took me thirty-one years to look at how and what I could do to be happy. And a part of my healing is sharing this story of pain and how I made it through. This part of my life was awful, disparaging, and intense. I am here to tell the world that those events have not defined me, and I have found healthy avenues to express myself. It is never too late to change and to heal.

I have recaptured my spirit of partaking in healthy adventures. I am a seeker of knowledge and extremely resilient. I have fostered healthy relationships and healthy activities. I am an artist, and my art is healing. Each day I create to express my emotions. I no longer push my feelings down because I know it is a dangerous thing for me. Art does heal! I find a flow and a peaceful zone within my art creations.

I am now married to an incredibly supportive man who loves me for me! My professional and personal lives are now ONE. I finally love me!

I am a determined, irresistible woman of my word living a stellar life!

Reflection:

Have you ever been in a situation where you had to make a split-second decision for your safety? Reflecting on this would you do anything differently?

If you had a friend in a similar situation, how would you support her?

Have you ever been traumatized? If so, what did you do to heal?

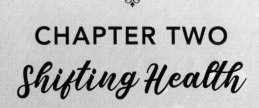

CHAPTER TWO
Shifting Health

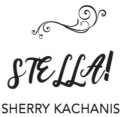

STELLA!

SHERRY KACHANIS

*A*fter being cancer-free for seven months, I requested to meet with my surgeon to discuss a colostomy reversal. At the appointment, he discussed the advantages, disadvantages, preparation protocol, and post-protocol before agreeing to schedule a surgery date, depending upon the results of my colonoscopy and PET scan.

As scan day approached, I had racing thoughts and was not breathing deeply—sure signs that I felt anxious and off-center about the pending results. I breathed deeply, inhaling for a count of seven, held for seven, and then released for seven. I repeated this pattern seven times. This practice brings me back into my body and allows me to feel calm. Meditation also helped. Despite doing breathing exercises and meditating, I still felt uneasy; something did not feel right.

Healthwise, I felt great! I walked two to three miles several times a week, ate clean and well, listened to healing and happy music, meditated, and spent hours playing in the gardens daily. Every day, I counted my blessings! In many ways, I had taken life for granted, as if I had an unlimited number of tomorrows.

The initial surgery left me with a colostomy. In the beginning,

41

I had difficulty accepting the colostomy. Having a colostomy kicked the living daylights out of my self-esteem, self-confidence, and self-image. I felt disconnected from myself. I knew it was why I had survived and felt gratitude, yet I did not love it. To foster a connection, I named her Stella. Whenever I felt sad or fearful, I cried out, "STELLA!" like in the movie *A Streetcar Named Desire.* I'd giggle and feel better.

Before the surgery, I knew nothing about colostomies, ostomies, or stomas. At first, it was overwhelming, yet as time passed, I became more comfortable with Stella. I was hyperaware of the colostomy bag and worried that everyone could see the outline of it under my clothes. I could see it, so I felt others could too. My husband, Stewart, reminded me that I see it because I knew it was there, while no one else did. I wondered if I would ever feel sexy again. As my body healed, I gained weight, and I grappled with having a bag at my midline. None of this helped my overall self-image.

After the cancer diagnosis, having PET scans quarterly became the norm and routine as part of the oncology care plan. When scan day arrived, I felt calm and relaxed because I meditated before the appointment. I listened to meditative music while waiting for the radioactive sugar to activate in my body. While in the PET scan machine, I asked myself if the cancer had returned. I felt a resounding *yes* in my body. Deep down, I knew.

I saw the oncologist later in the week to get the results. Stewart felt we had nothing to be concerned with; I was healing and finally regaining stamina. I told him something was off, yet he brushed it aside, thinking I was anxious. I slept poorly the night before the appointment. Exhausted and nervous, I meditated before seeing the doctor.

After the usual pleasantries with the doctor, he got right to the point—the cancer had returned. Even though I was mentally prepared, I immediately went numb, and tears started to flow uncontrollably from my eyes. The thought of chemo physically made me nauseous, and everything in my being said *no*. After the first surgery, I declined chemo after seven different tests returned a unanimous negative response for cancer. My husband supported my decision even though he would have chosen differently for himself. At that time, we agreed that I would do things my way. If something changed, then I would consider chemo.

Stewart asked the doctor questions. I am so grateful for his incredible advocacy because while I was physically present, mentally, I'd checked out. I was aware enough to tell the doctor I needed a day or two to process the information before deciding our course of action. As the news sank into my consciousness, the tears continued flowing.

On the drive home, I quietly sobbed. When we got home, my husband wanted to talk, but I did not. I could not. Fear, anger, sadness, and disappointment flowed through me fast and furiously. I went into my room to meditate, pray, and ask God for assistance and guidance about what path was best for my healing. While meditating, I asked myself, "What do I still need to learn from this cancer experience that once I learn and understand, I will be cancer-free?"

Stewart knew I was grappling with this recurrence. While I meditated, he called our mentor and friend to request that he talk with me. My husband quietly entered the room, waited for me to open my eyes, and handed me his phone. Our friend asked how I was doing, what I felt, and what I feared most. It was a deep discussion, going to the core of my fears. I was grateful for the conversation, as it gave me clarity on what I must do. The rest of the day, I let myself feel the emotions as they surfaced. I cried, sobbed, screamed, wrote, meditated, and prayed. Eventually, I came back to gratitude, especially how grateful I was to be alive. 43

The next day, Stewart and I discussed what to do. We decided that I would do whatever it took to be well, including chemo. Chemo wasn't something I wanted to experience; my stomach churned just hearing the word. Before starting chemo, I talked with a friend who shared the experience of having a colostomy. I told her I struggled with having chemo.

She suggested reframing the way I viewed chemo, as mindset is everything. Instead of seeing it as something negative, she recommended I see it as a magical elixir, flowing into me to eradicate abnormal and cancerous cells. I loved this, for it shifted my perspective of seeing chemo as something positive rather than negative.

Chemo is delivered in cycles. My first day of the first cycle was long and arduous. Almost immediately afterward, nausea struck, and, without much warning, I vomited, followed by dry heaves that lasted more than eight hours. I barely ate because of the queasiness. By late Saturday night, I was running a low-grade fever. Stewart called the on-call doctor, who advised taking ibuprofen or acetaminophen for the low-grade fever and asked us to check in the following day.

The next morning when my husband called, he was told to take me to the hospital's emergency room. They checked me out in the ER, gave me fluids for dehydration, and sent me home. I was a hot mess. I felt terrible, and my spirits were waning.

That night I looked at Stewart and said, "Honey, I do not know if I can do this."

He asked, "Do what?"

I said, "Chemo."

He looked at me and said, "Babe, you got this. I know it is hard, yet you are strong and will get through it."

I appreciated his encouragement, yet I felt simultaneously exhausted, angry, and sad.

A few days later, while talking with a friend, she reminded
me of the importance of surrender, as in letting go, to be in the moment of now and nowhere else. She gently reminded me that I was resisting the process, and resistance was making things more painful than necessary. She was right. From then on out, I committed to going into each chemo session with the attitude that

I was there to spread love and light to all. I would still be me, whether I was on a cancer journey or not. Once I let go, I flowed through each cycle with ease and grace.

While this chapter continues, with twists and turns, I still believe that one day I will hear the words, "Sherry, you are cancer-free!"

Reflection:

Have you or a friend ever received a scary medical diagnosis? What tools did you leverage to work through your feeling and experience?

How does resistance show up in your life? Do you lean in or push resistance away? How does this serve you?

Think of a time when you received bad news. How did you respond and how would you have liked to respond?

The Lightning Strike

MARY BETH GUDEWICZ

*I*n my usual haste, I felt the need to jump in the car and get my mom's new dog a toy the day before we were going to drive back home. My daughter, who had just the day before graduated college, wanted to go with me.

As my daughter and I drove out of the neighborhood, I heard my daughter scream, "Mom look out!"

I looked out of the left corner of my eye, and I saw a large truck barreling at us. I braced for impact as I turned the wheel and felt the punch of the truck as it slammed into our car. It felt as if I got slammed back into my body, and I could hear my daughter's voice.

"Mom, are you okay? Mom, are you okay?" she said, screaming and sobbing at the same time.

I felt liquid running down into my hands. When I looked down, my hands were covered in blood. I turned to look at my daughter.

She was dialing 911, saying, "My mom's head is bleeding. I don't know if she is okay."

I felt around my head and didn't notice any gashes or gaping wounds. I asked my daughter, "Are you okay?"

"I'm fine," she said between hiccupping sobs.

I took an inventory of my body and noticed my right knee felt a little sore, blood was on my shirt and pants but, overall, I felt completely calm and clear. I stepped out of the car, and my right leg gave out. I had to sit on the curb and wait for the paramedics to assist me onto the bed to be loaded into the ambulance.

As I sat in the ambulance with this sense of calmness and presence, I watched the numbers tick up on the digital clock inside the ambulance. At 14:43:12, a loud voice came into my right ear, "This is your lightning strike."

The next week and a half, I remember as clear as day. In the emergency room, I discovered I had fractured my tibia plateau. They stented me immediately, saying I needed to get into surgery ASAP. I remembered the drive home from Kansas, sitting in the back seat of our truck, my leg propped as I called orthopedic surgeons, hoping one could fit me in immediately. My whole focus was on how quickly I could heal my physical body.

My ability to laser focus on the problem at hand came from living my life, always fighting for my place. For example, when I started playing volleyball, I couldn't even hit a ball over the net and didn't make the high school freshman team. I practiced every day on the side of the house, working my way to making the high school sophomore volleyball team, playing open ball during the offseason, junior varsity the next year, and varsity my senior year with an offer to play in college. My physical healing was viewed in that same systematic way: this is what I need to do, and I will meet the goals of walking, playing golf, and resuming my normal activities sooner than what I was told. My superhero, against-all-odds personality came out that summer.

My physical healing progressed quickly thanks to my anti-inflammatory diet, visualization exercises, weight lifting, and daily meditation. I continued running my business since it was virtual and worked on my physical healing. I spent a lot of time letting everything go except for my healing and my client work. I relearned to walk in less than three months after surgery. I was right on target when the next strike hit.

I started having these intense dreams and moments in my daily life where everything felt different. As if the life I knew was starting to shift. There were things I liked to do that I did not want to do anymore. I couldn't tolerate violence in any form. I felt lost in my world. Then I remembered the words in the ambulance, "This is your lightning strike."

I knew these words were my signal to take the advice I gave to my clients to look deeper. I have always been an open-minded person, studying energy from how it works with the physical body through each mental, emotional, and spiritual layer. I took a step back and looked deeper into the next steps of my healing journey. It went back to what "This is your lightning strike" meant.

My accident sent me on a trajectory of taking stock of where I was, how committed I was to heal on all levels, and how ready I was to step into the next phase of my life's journey. My work involved marrying science with spirituality. I faced with working through these deeper levels to truly heal. I knew this, and I also felt a bit lost with a tad of dread thrown in.

I kept asking, "Am I ready and willing to do the work?" I sat and listened to myself, and then I knew. To truly move on in my life, I needed to do the work immediately and face my demon that had been at the root of my choices, such as how I acted with people, how I trusted, and being in alignment with my soul.

I sought the help of mentors to start this next-level healing. I examined patterns in my life, starting with my family of origin, school relationships, coaches, bosses, and business associates. I realized there was one underlying core belief of myself that was a pattern in all of those relationships: I had a deep fear of rejection. This core belief defined every choice in my life and created this need to push myself, prove myself worthy, self-sabotage, and keep myself closed off so I wouldn't get hurt. But I still got hurt, and this pattern continued to keep me on the hamster wheel that I just wanted to get off. This was my lightning strike.

51

This realization caused a floodgate to open within me. I felt pressure in my chest and tears streaming down my face—all indications that I had hit upon my truth. I had a choice: do I heal that part of me, or do I acknowledge it and move on? In my heart, I knew I needed to do the work to align myself with my soul. I couldn't hide any longer or pretend. My lightning strike was healing this core belief of fear of rejection to be my authentic self and live in alignment with my soul.

Now, a year after the accident, I am still working on healing my core belief. Have I made strides? Absolutely! Is my work complete? No. That is okay because true healing for me has never been a simple road. But the freeing aspect is knowing how to heal these wounds on a mental, emotional, and spiritual level, and each day is a step closer to being in alignment with my soul. I feel more whole now than I did a year ago, and that is how I know I am healing.

Reflection:

What has been a lightning strike moment in your life? Did you discover what needed to change or be healed? Did you do the work? How is your life now?

When you evaluate your life, what continuing patterns do you notice? What can you do to shift those patterns? Journal your discoveries.

Has your life become so busy you aren't listening? If so, what can you let go of in your schedule to make the time to listen? Why are you keeping yourself busy? When you stop and listen this week, what is your body, mind and spirit telling you?

Decision Point

FELICIA MESSINA-D'HAITI

I had been here before, wearing a similar blue gown, waiting for the doctor to enter the room. I had already read the pathology report and had the preliminary phone call asking me to come in to discuss the results and treatment plan with the doctor. While this was a new experience, it was also a bit too familiar. The doctor greeted me as he entered the room with somewhat of an apology that we are meeting again under *these* circumstances. As we discussed the pathology report in detail, I experienced feelings of deep disappointment and frustration.

In the previous seven years, I had experienced two different cancer diagnoses. The first was advanced-stage colon cancer; the second was early-stage breast cancer. Moving through each of those journeys, I went through a myriad of emotions. Through it all, though, I remained hopeful that they would only be a blip on my life's journey, and I would move on being in better health. I do admit that I was much more hopeful after the first diagnosis than after the second. With the second diagnosis, it took me longer to shift into a more positive mindset. And here we were again where suspicious cells were confirmed to be cancerous.

I was full of questions. *Was this a recurrence, or a new occurrence?*

How had this happened after the previous cancer was removed? How had it happened after I had radiation treatments in the same area? I felt angry. What had been the point of the radiation? It obviously hadn't worked. And then there was the journey with endocrine therapy. I was already on my third different kind of therapy because the side effects from the first two had been debilitating. I felt like I had been through enough. Disappointment gave way to confusion.

While the doctors expressed confidence that the lumpectomy removed the cancerous area, their recommendation for the next step was a single mastectomy. After the first diagnosis, I was told that the chance of recurrence or new cancers forming was less than 10 percent, and less than 5 percent with the support of the endocrine therapy. Yet, here I was facing this new choice, and I felt resistant and bewildered, trying to make sense of it all. Was this really necessary? It seemed so extreme to me. After all, the surgeon said he removed the cancer, right? Yet, because I had radiation treatments in that same area just a year ago, I would not be able to undergo those treatments again. Despite the completion of the previous treatment plan, new cancers formed so the treatment plan had to be different this time.

I struggled with these questions for what felt like an eternity. In reality, it was about six weeks. I was definitely, without a doubt, resistant to the new treatment plan. I emailed the doctors a million questions about other treatment options and percentages of recurrence. I appreciated their patience. They answered every question. They wanted me to be comfortable with whatever decision I made and gave me time to process it all, which frankly reinforced my questions about the urgency of it. At one point, I wondered how long I could drag out the decision process because I just simply was not ready to make a choice. The doctors explained that scheduling a surgery date when the two doctors were available might be challenging, so I scheduled a date a few months out, "just in case."

During this time of decision-making, I was scheduled for my yearly mammogram. Since the first diagnosis, I had an annual mammogram and another diagnostic mammogram that focused on the previous cancer area. Before each test, I experienced some anxiety, though the more I became aware of my own patterns of running down a rabbit hole of despair, I could stop, take a breath, and pray to realign my energy.

The technician took photos, sent them electronically to the doctor, then we waited for a response to determine if I could get dressed and leave or if they needed additional images. I certainly was not surprised when the technician said that the doctor wanted ed more images of an area of concern. What shocked me was that, for the first time ever, this area of concern was in my left breast, which had never had any issues at all.

After the pictures were taken, I dressed and got ready to leave. The technician ushered me to a separate room to have a video chat with the radiologist. During that meeting, the doctor explained what I had already heard multiple times: there was a suspicious area for which they wanted to biopsy the cells. I made the appointment for the following month. And again, I anxiously waited for the results to pop up in my medical portal. And when they did, I was both relieved and troubled—relieved because they did not find cancerous cells, yet troubled because they did find atypical cells that brought my mind directly back to the times in the year or two prior to the diagnosis where similar cells were found on the right side.

Suddenly, my decision-making process shifted from whether or not I should have a single mastectomy to deciding if I wanted a double mastectomy. I prayed, meditated, reflected, did research, and emailed the surgeon all of my questions. This time, he called to answer all of my questions and to say that he understood my reasoning, reassuring me that it was my decision. It was my desire (and still is) to be as healthy as possible and also to be free of the monitoring and apprehension about the scans. It was at that point that I chose to not only confirm the surgery but to shift the procedure to a double mastectomy.

After the surgery, the pathology report described cancerous cells found in both breasts. And though this had been a major surgery with some complications that currently I am healing from and learning how to move forward, I've already had some significant insights about the path of my journey and how I was processing it and making decisions.

What struck me most was my delayed decision-making. I had been living in limbo, fence sitting, not wanting to commit to either side. Upon reflection, I now see that I had done that in other areas of my life since my first cancer diagnosis. I waited to make decisions, not committing to any choice, not defining or expressing my desires. With many things, I simply went with the flow and dealt with whatever the resulting experience was. To me, it was as if I had stopped steering the boat on my journey because I wasn't quite sure if I would still be here to reach my goals or desired outcomes.

It was as if I floated aimlessly, testing all of the waters instead of jumping in at any point and then resetting if I needed to. This lack of decision-making led to a lack of commitment to my goals, a lack of being "all in" on anything for fear of more disappointment or more sadness. When looking back, I feel that these patterns were fairly obvious, but I could not see them in the moment. Now, I am more ready to dive in and just make a decision, choose something. Anything. If it turns out that I made a choice that I don't like, I have the option to make a new choice at any time and still be 100 percent committed to that choice. The judgments I held about whether something was a good experience or not are just that—my own judgments. Everything I experience is what I make of it, and I know that choices I make with positive expectancy will always turn out better than the experience of simply floating around, waiting for the winds to push me in a new direction and still not fully making a choice.

While experiencing even a single cancer diagnosis, or any un-expected life-altering situation, was not something that I would willingly choose, I treasure what I have learned about myself through these three different cancer experiences. And I under-stand that no matter what choices I make in my life, committing to them with determination and positive expectancy will allow me to live my life with greater joy.

Reflection:

How would you view your life if you see every experience as a conscious choice?

Where can you find the treasures in challenging experiences?

How can commitment to your choices create magical life experiences?

The Body Knows

MICHELLE LEMOI

A single tear rolled down my face as the breathing machine hummed. I was sick … again. The wheezing in my left lung was a constant reminder that I had overdone it. Again. I was frightened. This never used to happen. This wheezing in my left lung was new. New to the last couple of times I've been sick. I didn't like it.

I'm blessed with the ability to go, go, go. As a woman working in the construction industry, I've pushed myself to extreme limits for the last thirty years. Being surrounded by all that masculine energy of doing, pushing, and striving is like running on auto-pilot. Fifty-plus hour weeks working at top speed means most days I ran on adrenaline. Additionally, I'm a single mom spending time with my child while fitting in networking and working on my business. I wore my achievements and ability to conquer all like a badge of honor.

I'm a healthy individual with a strong immune system, so when I get sick, it's a big deal. I fall hard and for a long period of time. But with the first symptoms, I push, ignore, and power through.

The first prolonged bout of sickness happened in December of 2012. I had just returned from a vacation. Three days after getting back from the trip, I had immense congestion, and it began leaking into my lungs. I increased my inhalers, took a cold and sinus medication, a cough syrup, and kept going. I was running my business, running a household, and it was almost Christmas. There was NO time to be sick.

But by Christmas, I could barely stand. I couldn't find any time to rest, and my lungs sounded terrible. I was hopeful that I could rest during Christmas break. In the meantime, I started toting my breathing machine with me to the office, ensuring I did my treatments every four hours. I'd seen my pulmonologist, and he prescribed a course of steroids.

By early January, there was no change. I returned to the doctor and was administered a shot of steroids. By the time I walked out of his office, I could breathe. Within a matter of days, I was back to my normal self.

I did not learn my lesson.

This happened again in 2019 around Thanksgiving. I went through three courses of oral steroids, breathing treatments, and a visit to a different pulmonologist. I spent New Year's Eve in the hospital. I couldn't breathe. That was the first time I heard the wheezing in my left lung. What was happening?

By the second week in January, I desperately called the practice begging for help and was seen by a new pulmonologist. He shared with me my body was in a "sick loop." What?!

I left his office armed with an arsenal of medication and prescriptions. I had a piece of paper with an hourly regimen of what I needed to do to get better. Within two weeks, I felt relief. Three weeks later, the wheezing in my lungs had ceased.

I gained twenty pounds from all the steroids, and my body was exhausted.

I hadn't missed one day of work.

It would be another three years before I was sick again.

In December 2022, I had been working fifty-plus hours again, consulting part-time, and I was teaching a workshop at a construction company.

Three days before the workshop, I began to feel the bone-weary exhaustion, the intermittent congestion, the hoarse voice, and the tightening lungs. There was NO time to be sick. I convinced myself I was healthier than before. I knew I would rest during Christmas break. I could make it.

Except I didn't.

I successfully completed the workshop, but as I slid into the seat of the car for the drive home, I knew I was in trouble. I'd pushed it again, and what followed was another seven weeks of being ill.

This time, I knew I had to do things differently. I rested. I canceled everything on my schedule. I took a couple of days off from work, and I sat still my entire holiday vacation. I slept, drank lots of water, did my breathing treatments every four hours, and took another round of steroids.

But the biggest shift came from sitting still. I realized in those moments that I'm uncomfortable with doing nothing. It feels strange. My brain goes into overdrive with all the things I should be doing. I get anxious and panicky.

Yet my body and the Universe were sending me a clear message. You need to stop and rest. You must learn this lesson. You cannot continually push your body to its limits like you have been.

Consciously and logically, I know this. But I would NOT under any circumstances allow it.

Why? Because all the pushing, doing, and striving was tied to my worth. My worth as a person. If I wasn't doing all the things, then who was I? What was I here for? Was there a reward in doing nothing? Am I supposed to be still?

I felt guilty. I felt like I wasn't allowed to rest. What would people think of me? I realized I had no compassion for myself when I was sick. I was holding myself to some unsustainable standard that was an old story I learned from my childhood.

What I needed was radical change. I received pushback not just from myself but from others. People were so used to me pushing

65

through, so setting a boundary that I came first in order to get my health back on track was abnormal.

It meant doing the bare minimum in my life. It meant doing everything to get better and all the while listening to that wheezing in my left lung. That scary sound when I inhaled and exhaled and wondered, "Why the left side only? Why is this now the go-to symptom, and what does that mean for the future?"

A trip to the pulmonologist after vacation revealed my lungs were clear with no issues on a chest x-ray. But the warning he gave was clear. "You cannot push yourself like this. You have to recognize the symptoms earlier and rest in order to heal. The medicine helps, but only rest lets the body heal."

I was heartbroken. I realized I'd been abusing my body. I was embarrassed and ashamed to know that I had ignored the symptoms, the messages, and the signs that my body was sending to me because life was demanding and more important.

I set out to change the story. I needed to shift from those masculine energies of pushing, doing, and striving and embrace being, resting, and receiving—my feminine essence. It's not the popular path, but it's the only path if I want to discontinue causing myself harm.

Embracing rest and stillness, I would curl up on the sofa with my blanket and spend hours lying there, reading historical fiction and sleeping. I'd journal when negative emotions flared or when my brain was in overdrive thinking about what I wasn't doing or accomplishing. I used EFT tapping to calm my body and tell it that this new way was safe and that I deserved this time of healing. I had to do the work to disrupt the old way of being.

As I gained my strength, I realized the challenge was going to be how to manage this new way as I jumped back into life. It's not easy for me. It's a practice.

I try to limit what I say yes to. I assess my energy and health levels on a daily basis. I ensure I'm adding regular fun to my life. I sleep in and nap often. I get to bed every night at the same time.

I drink lots of water. When I'm feeling sick, I stop and check in with my body. What does it need?

Life isn't stopping, but I can slow it down. My goal is to never hear that wheezing again. That sound is the ultimate scare. I acknowledge and vow to take pristine care of myself.

I have only one magnificent body in this precious lifetime. It's time to connect fully with it and take care of it as I would anything else in my life. No longer can I come last. I'm hoping the Universe and my body will be happy I've learned my lesson.

Reflection:

In what ways do you appreciate your health? Are there changes you've wanted to make to improve your health, but haven't? What's one step you could take now to make that shift?

When your brain is in overdrive, what tools do you use to change gears?

How does your body give you clues that you ought to rest and recover? Do you listen or push through?

CHAPTER THREE
Shifting Relationships

Waking Beauty

ROSA MARIA SZYNSKI

There was nothing remarkable to me about that night. I tucked in my two little boys after saying prayers with them. I wrote in my journal, and, as usual, I said my own prayers, expressing gratitude for the things I had, never asking for anything more except the protection of my loved ones and peace in my heart to sleep well. Soon, I drifted off to sleep.

My dream was more real to me than anything I had ever experienced in my waking hours. I was sitting next to a man in a car, and we were talking. I felt like he was right there, like I could touch him. And I did. We were together, a couple. We shared a tender kiss, and then soon after the kiss, the dream ended, or I woke up. I lay in the dark, turning the dream around in my head, wondering what it meant.

That morning, I walked around in a daze, and the only thing I can clearly remember from that day is how I sat on the floor and flipped through old yearbook pages looking for clues. At one point, I saw his picture, and I absolutely knew it was the boy in my dream.

He had written, "You made those days the most memorable days of my life. I know I probably haven't said everything I wanted to say, but what we leave behind is not lost. I wish you a happiness that will last a lifetime."

I had not seen Gregg in twenty-one years, since the day of our high school graduation, but I read those words every once in a while whenever I packed up my things to move. On that day, however, I read them as though seeing them for the first time. At eighteen, his heartfelt wishes for my life were laced with an awareness that our time had come to an end but that he would remain a part of me and I a part of him. We never dated, yet he was by my side for two of the biggest events of my high school career. We were connected in a way that didn't require us to spend lots of time getting to know one another.

Gregg was almost literally the boy next door. He lived down the street from me ever since I moved into my new neighborhood in fifth grade. We never talked until high school. He was extremely shy, and I was never quite able to express what I truly wanted to say. Our teacher assigned him as my biology lab partner in our one and only class together in four years. After that, I gathered up the courage to approach him and ask if he would be my escort when I was nominated for both junior prom and senior basketball homecoming courts. Each time, he said yes, and each time he accompanied me, I won.

Still mesmerized by my dream but a little more aware of what was happening around me, I went to work the next day and began to prepare the lesson materials for my kindergarten class. I turned on my computer, left the classroom to make copies, and returned when it was booted up. Then I sat down to check emails for important information. What I saw next seemed impossible. I was stunned. One email stood out to me, glaringly. There in the subject line was the name of the boy I just dreamed about. How could this be?

I sat for a few moments in bewilderment. *What was this dream about? Was something wrong? Why would Gregg's brother be writing to me after all these years if everything was fine? Why would he write to me at all? How did he find me? He hardly knew me. It's been twen-ty-one years!* When I finally opened the message that came from Gregg's brother, I saw it was a simple request. "This message is intended for Rosa. If it reaches the wrong person, please delete and accept my apology. Your name was brought up in conversations about old high school friends. Please reply if you're interested in getting in contact with Gregg. No reply means no thanks ..." The email was time-stamped shortly after the time of my dream.

I was not only the right Rosa, but I was the one who just had a dream about the very person he was referring to, the one I hadn't seen in over twenty-one years. By responding to the email, I said *yes* to the invitation and, when a few days passed and I didn't hear back, I knew something had changed. Gregg's father had unexpectedly passed away.

In one of his last conversations with his father, Gregg, who had no children, vowed he would never marry a second time.

His father, however, shared a vision, "You will get married, she will be beautiful, and you will have children."

It was a few more weeks before Gregg and I met in person. Though I lived over two hundred miles from our hometown, I discovered that Gregg lived just a few short miles away. We continued to write to one another every single day. For so long, I kept the secrets of my hopes and dreams tucked neatly away on the pages of my journal. Now, I couldn't believe I was freely writing about those same hopes and dreams in my letters, including how I saw myself having a daughter.

When we finally met for dinner, we were seated at a table for two. The food came and went, but we remained for hours. At one point, I told him I could live in a cardboard box if I was happy. I saw him look at me as though I had just hung the moon. I suppose it was something that resonated with him. Maybe it was *his* dream to find someone who would live with him in a cardboard box. I smiled at the thought of it.

Later, I learned that on the night of my dream, Gregg and his

75

brother were out for dinner. His brother asked him if he would ever get married again, to which Gregg replied, "There's only one. Her name is Rosa, and she lived in our neighborhood."

It was amazing to realize that while I was dreaming of Gregg, he was speaking my name.

By this time, I was experiencing synchronicity and joy like nothing I had ever known in my whole life. These were the moments I was searching for, the ones I prayed about in my journal. This was also the moment I learned that both joy and sorrow could live side-by-side. Over the next days, weeks, and months, as I was falling in love with a new life, it became clear that it was time for me to leave my old one. I could not imagine how anyone exits one life to enter a completely new existence. Again, I prayed for direction in the pages of my journal.

Going through divorce was the hardest thing I ever did in my life. Most people didn't understand what I was experiencing, so it meant letting go of friendships, stepping back from family, and releasing the voices that implored me to wake up or I would look back in regret years later. What they didn't know was that I *was* awake and, while I had no way to see the future exactly, I felt as though I was being carried through each step by a beautiful peace-filled flow with no fear. For the first time in my life, I was trusting my journey.

Gregg and I were married the next year, and the year after that, the boys welcomed their baby sister, who we named Grace. It's been eighteen years since I woke up from my dream and began living in a world of dreams come true. I realize the difference between me *before* my dream and me *after* my dream has been my awareness and willingness to tune in, trust my heart, do what is aligned, and follow my dreams.

Reflection:

How has synchronicity shown up in your life? What does synchronicity mean to you?

Tell about a time when the joy of beginning something new coincided with the sorrow of ending or leaving something behind. What did you learn from the experience?

Is there a person from your past with whom you would like to reconnect? Describe what you would want that person to know about who you are now.

Answering God's Call

KAREN MCPHAIL

*T*he Parisian event had already begun. He came in late, and his coral-colored paisley shirt caught my eye. He exuded kindness. At our first break, I felt myself pulled toward him.

I opened the conversation, "How are you involved in this group?"

He explained he joined a business program, and the event had been an incentive for signing up for two years.

Suddenly, words flowed out of my mouth. "You will find the woman you are going marry."

As I heard these words, my brain was saying, *what are you doing?* Yet my words continued with authority and prophecy. "I couldn't help but notice you don't have a wedding ring on. You are going to find the woman you will marry in these programs. You have just made the best decision of your life!"

With that, I walked away, dazed. What had happened? What compelled me to do and say what I had?

The last night of the event, my retreat roommate, Liz, asked me if this same man, whose name was Doug, could join us for dinner.

We had a lovely dinner and then decided to go on an adventure to find Hemingway's home since Liz and I had been searching for it all week. We found it! We took a picture in front of the brilliant, cobalt-blue door. Another pleasant memory of Paris was made.

But why was I in Paris to begin with? What was highly improbable turned possible through a series of God moments, serendipities, and the kindness and generosity of others, which resulted in me having enough courage to attend this self-empowerment retreat in Paris—alone.

It started a year before. I sat drinking coffee in the dark of morning when I heard a loud voice from the corner of the otherwise empty room say, "You will create a program to give young teens and young adults HOPE."

Talk about a life-altering experience! Despite being a single mom with two kids and entirely unsure HOW I would do this, I told the principal at the elementary school where I taught that I would not be returning the following year. I would take a year's sabbatical to follow the Calling I had received from God.

Looking back now, I realize this was my first "YES" that activated the miraculous journey of all dots aligning in the Universe for me to meet my soulmate.

On my return from Paris, I went back to working on my master's degree, which was part of the Calling, and continued being a vessel for it.

This period was not without struggles. Two months after coming back from Paris, I ended a two-year relationship. I believe God presented a situation knowing it would end the relationship with no option for reconciliation.

Fear, doubt, and an array of insecurities surfaced. I came face-to-face with the reality that I might be alone for the rest of my life. I tried to stay in faith and prayed to God to bring me a man of his design, a man of the highest integrity.

Shortly, I would be an empty nester. My youngest child was starting his senior year, and my best friend, Tess, my yellow lab of thirteen years, was blind and aging.

I felt broken, alone, and uncertain of my future, especially regarding meeting a soulmate partner. Looking at my soulmate dream board, I contemplated whether my standards were too high. Maybe this guy didn't even exist! I pulled off the strip of fancy paper that read, "Sharp dresser, sense of style."

I threw it away, then caught myself. "This is a dream board! Don't you dare dial your dreams "down" to fit the mediocre reality you are experiencing!" I retrieved the paper and pasted it back on.

Soon after, I heard something from Joe Dispenza that moved my life in a different trajectory. He responded to the question, "How do we manifest a soulmate?" I'm paraphrasing, but what I took away from what I heard was: when you become the soulmate, you desire and love your life, and your vibrational frequency will draw that person to you.

I decided to become the soulmate I desired! It couldn't be a double standard … anything I desired him to be, I needed to be or become. My metamorphosis of becoming my own soulmate and loving the life I lived began.

A few months later, I had a huge setback when I believed the person I had started dating briefly might be "the one" and ended up not to be. This breakup shattered me.

I needed a counseling session for this one. When I came out of the session, I was even lower than when I went in. I felt childish having believed that soulmates existed.

I feared mentally going any lower as I was feeling deep despair. There was a lovely restaurant a block away. I took myself to lunch with hopes of shifting this disheartenment.

While eating, a voice note came from a Paris retreat participant. It had been eight months since the retreat. She explained that she just received a message from God that she was to tell me to contact Doug.

I said, "Doug from Paris?"

As she confirmed this, I asked if I could tell him she had given me this message. I had no idea what to say to Doug after so much time had passed. She said I was on my own; she had done her part by delivering the message.

I believe in Callings and divine messages. I took this information as absolute truth.

When I arrived home, I Facebook messaged Doug. I told him I craved conversation with him. We planned a call for two days later.

I watched the movie *Under the Tuscan Sun* that night and, coupled with the message I received about Doug earlier, I felt a new hope and excitement about my future.

On my first call with Doug, I chose to put it all out there. I told him about the Calling and how anyone in my life was going to have to be okay with what would unfold because of it.

His father had been a pastor for over fifty years. Doug was accustomed to this phenomenon, which further reinforced for me God's hand in this allowing me to trust and open my heart.

We had three-hour Zoom dates over the next few months before we booked a trip to meet face-to-face in San Francisco the last weekend in May.

The first weekend in May, I attended a conference in Denver with a girlfriend. The day before I left, Doug asked if he could have dinner with me that Saturday. I told him I wasn't bringing my computer.

He said, "Karen, you're only twelve hundred miles away from me ... I can't not fly in and have dinner with you."

That was the most romantic thing I had ever heard. Our dinner was amazing! I told my girlfriend I was going to marry him. I knew in my heart he was THE ONE!

Three weeks later, in San Francisco, we had a magical weekend with Doug proposing and putting a gorgeous ring on my finger! Two days later, I resigned from my teaching job.

My son graduated from high school and would be headed to college. Doug flew out to meet my son and daughter. Three weeks later, I went to Michigan to meet his family, and we got married while I was there!

He surprised me by flying out my son and daughter, as well as the beautiful soul who was God's messenger, to attend the wedding.

My Oregon house went on the market and sold while I was in Michigan. Everything flowed "divinely" as if a magic wand had been waved above us.

I came home and, over the next few weeks, finished my master's while packing my whole life into one POD.

Doug flew to Oregon for our second wedding. The next day, we left for the most spectacular Italian honeymoon imaginable.

Marrying my soulmate completely shifted every aspect of my life. This was God's plan, and I trusted it even when others around me thought I was crazy.

Michigan is our home until we decide where we'll go to fulfill our mutual passion for travel and adventure.

Saying "YES" to God, to loving life, and to myself empowered me to live my happily ever after.

Reflection:

Reflect on a time that you received intuitive information and acted upon it. What happened?

Have you ever had a "Divine download" that led you to take inspired action? How did you receive the information and what happened?

In what areas of your life can you increase your "yes" responses? Where can you say "no" more frequently?

The Wounds of Betrayal

YVETTE LEFLORE

I was exhausted, mentally and emotionally. I felt like I was spinning in circles. For the past few years, I had been building my energy practice alongside the hustle business I had had for twenty-five years. I knew how to make the hustle work, but it wore me down. My energy practice filled me with peace, and I felt compelled to grow it, but I could not fully commit. At the dinner table, I frequently shared my struggles, and my husband would patiently look at me and say, "You've been having this conversation for a long time."

The biggest stumbling block to releasing the hustle in favor of the energy-healing practice was that I lacked confidence that I could generate enough income to contribute to our household. My husband suggested that I allow him to take care of the bills so I could thrive in a place that would nourish me. That would have been great, but the deeply ingrained messages from my youth of "you need to provide for yourself and never trust a man" had the upper hand. From the ages of four through seventeen, I experienced three men exiting my life, leaving my mother to financially support our family.

At times I shared with friends a vision of growing my energy practice and leaving the hustle. I'd ask questions like "Who would I be without this twenty-five-year career defining me? Could I make it work?" The feedback I received was a mixed bag. Some offered tepid encouragement when I shared my dreams while others were unabashedly enthusiastic.

I took classes, gained clients, and experienced some traction with my energy practice only to look at the overwhelming reality of what stood before me and run back to the safety of the hustle. Not only was I lured by the money but also the success. I wasn't comfortable in the unknown that the energy practice represented. The success and safety of the known were intoxicating and grounding.

Then my husband got a new job, and we moved to a new state that significantly decreased our cost of living. *What excuses did I have with money no longer my main concern and a husband who kept encouraging me to follow my dreams? Was it time to take that leap of faith and answer my soul's call?*

For the first year in the new house, the room that I claimed as my energy work haven—my spirit room—lay dormant. It contained a storage closet for things that were not needed daily, and each time I walked through the spirit room to retrieve something I heard the room whisper to me. I felt peace as I looked out the French doors to the woods and saw birds at the feeders. The room enveloped me with love. My spirit guides and ancestors asked me to get settled in the room and reconnect with my energy practice.

"I'm not ready yet," I said as I left the room, chagrined and full of self-judgment, unable to answer that call.

After a year in our new area, as I scrolled Facebook, I discovered a local group that offered a weekly spiritual growth and meditation class. It was the first time since our arrival that I had seen anything like it. Believing there are no accidents, I saw this as a sign from the spirits, and I felt pulled to go.

By the end of the first meeting, I was in tears. I realized I had found my spiritual home in my new state. Not only did I connect with this like-minded group of women, but I also learned this area had a large community of healers. The embers of my energy business slowly started to reignite. Once again, I declared myself an energy healer. I connected with people of similar beliefs, finally spent time in my spirit room, and reclaimed my space in the energy-healing business world.

Although I was growing my energy practice, I still felt myself drowning in indecision. The safety of a business I had run for over a quarter of a century strangled my joy as I still felt beholden to creating an income, all while knowing it would take time to grow a financially viable energy practice.

As I lamented, my ever-patient husband pushed at me to follow my heart, and I pushed back saying I couldn't do that; I was not ready to give up my income from the other business. What I did not say out loud was I needed to know I could support myself because nothing is ever for sure.

One night he pushed back harder. "I don't think you are ready to allow someone to take care of you; it's something you've never permitted."

I felt the air rush from my lungs, tears filled my eyes, and my throat closed. I was speechless. Fear gripped me. *Allow myself to be taken care of? Permit a MAN to provide?* It went against everything I had been taught.

Unfortunately, the tendrils of "don't trust a man" had firmly wrapped themselves around my base chakra—the center for safety and security—and my money center. Their grip created scar tissue and adhesions that had grown stronger every time I was betrayed. I had work to do to heal those wounds. I suddenly understood THIS is what I had been fighting these many years.

This inner conversation about money was a riptide that kept pulling me under, and I, a panicked swimmer, exerted all my energy fighting against it. Then I remembered that if caught in a riptide, the best thing a swimmer can do is release the panic and swim parallel to the shore. As my panic about money dissipated,

89

my body released its tension allowing me to tap into my intuition.

My intuition led me to heal and grow in many ways over the next months. I enrolled in a program and learned how to work with the energy of the elements. I meditated, connected with my ancestors, journaled, worked with spiritual teachers, and received energy work.

While all this was happening, my husband and I experienced the fruits of my hustle business—an earned trip to Puerto Rico. While sitting at the bar with my favorite sales manager from the company I repped, a warm breeze blowing, music thrumming, and a cold beverage in hand, I declared, for the first time, "I'm stepping away from my leadership role in this business." I cried and told her I did not know when, but I knew it was coming. I shared how the leadership role was no longer feeding my soul; in fact, I felt like it was starving.

Once I made my declaration, I created an exit plan. I deepened my involvement with the metaphysical community in my area and took classes to add to my healing toolbox. I got my name out as a local healer and grew my distant client base. With each step forward, I felt the air fill my lungs and experienced a renewed sense of energy. I could breathe again, and I knew I was on the right path.

Just four months later, despite my trepidation, I retired from my leadership role in that company. Each time I questioned my direction and felt myself slipping back to safety, I utilized meditation, took a salt bath, or used one of my many tools to reconnect with my soul's call. Although I retired from my leadership role, I did not retire from selling; I still loved that part of the business. I got to let go of the need to rely on the hustle to provide the income. A sense of peace was omnipresent.

Just as I eased into this transition, my husband was diagnosed with lung cancer, news that rocked our world. It had the potential to reopen the wounds and allow the fear and "another man is leaving me" tendrils to take hold. I knew I had healed many of the scars when my thoughts were no longer about rebuilding my hustle business to make the money for safety and security but about continuing to grow my energy-healing practice and being the best healing partner for my husband. I had freed myself from most of the tendrils and made the shift. I had changed the conversation.

Reflection:

In what ways are you a natural leader in your life and career? How do you show appreciation to yourself for this leadership?

Have you ever moved to a new state or country, having to build new relationships? What worked for you? What would you do differently?

In what ways have your stumbling blocks transformed into foundation stones for your growth?

This Is the Man You're Going to Marry

LEE MURPHY WOLF

I didn't know if it was the rum punch talking or maybe the mushroom tea, but I found myself on my knees. Sinking into the sand, hands raised toward the moonlit sky, I screamed at the top of my lungs, "I can't do this anymore!"

Tears flowed down my cheeks, disintegrating into my skin and merging with the humid night air. I fell over and curled up into a tight ball.

I was completely alone. And I would be for the rest of my life.

I sat back up and quietly wiped the sand off my face. It was over. I was not going to try and make things work with Steve anymore.

A few minutes earlier, I spilled my guts to a total stranger. What started as small talk between two people on holiday became a series of true confessions.

I told him that I had come to the British Virgin Islands to put space between me and my boyfriend.

On the outside, things looked great. I had a smart, talented guy who adored me. But I was miserable on the inside. We were good friends and coworkers but completely incompatible as a couple. Our lifestyles, our dreams, and our values were so different. Three years later, my relationship—and my life—was a mess.

I showed this stranger the diamond ring I had just bought. It was an idea I got from Oprah. It symbolized my commitment to myself, a reminder not to settle in life.

After rambling on for what seemed like an eternity, I paused and asked, "What should I do?"

The stranger said, "You already made your decision. You just need to tell him."

That was not what I wanted to hear. I wanted a magic solution. I wanted to wave a wand and have Steve be exactly how I wanted him to be. I didn't want to be the "bad guy" and break it off.

But who was I kidding? The truth was I had been here before. I was almost forty years old and had a lousy track record in relationships.

My liaisons were predictable: guys who were full of potential but stuck in a cycle of addiction and affliction. Or guys who came with complex baggage and were not emotionally available.

Steve fell into the first category. He was creative and brilliant, doing everything in his power to dull himself just to get through life. And I was in a codependent loop, cycling between trying to fix him, being complacent, getting angry, and then shutting down.

What was wrong with me? Other people had "normal" relationships; why not me? Maybe my standards were too high. Or maybe I was selfish.

Things had gone too far with Steve. I was tired and had to accept that I was fighting for a relationship that was going nowhere and that if I didn't leave now, I would wind up like my parents.

A few days later, I was back in New York City, heading to a work function. A group of us were in a van, heading uptown.

"Your hair looks sunkissed," my colleague Mark said. He had a big grin on his face and was as enthusiastic as an overgrown puppy.

I groaned on the inside and replied, "Yeah, I just got back from vacation."

I continued to look straight ahead, concentrating on the back of the driver's seat. I wished my gaze could transport me back to the beach. I wanted to be left alone. I had a big problem and needed to sort out how I was going to break it off with my boyfriend.

Mark kept talking. He was so damn perky, like a ray of effin' sunshine.

"Can I tell you a joke?" he asked.

"I hate jokes," I thought to myself. But since there was nowhere else for me to go, I turned toward him and found myself saying, "Sure."

Why on earth did I say that? Total people-pleaser move. Ugh.

He begins, "Little Johnny is in third grade ..."

As I politely listened, his words washed over me like a gentle wave. I started feeling lighter, like I was floating out of my body. I could hear what he was saying, and yet his voice sounded far away, as if I was on a phone line that was underwater.

As he delivered the punchline, I heard a man's voice in my left ear, as clear as day, which is impossible because that was the ear by the window. And there was no one sitting behind me.

The voice, in a thick French accent, blurted out, rather abruptly, "This is the man you're going to marry."

Suddenly everything slowed down, almost to a standstill. The only thing I could see was Mark right in front of me. An aura of bright white light surrounded him. His blue eyes turned into kaleidoscopes, revealing an array of beautiful colors, shapes, and patterns.

I felt a wave of warmth move through me. And in that moment, I knew it was true.

"Oh my god ... this is the man I'm going to marry," I heard myself say inside my head.

The revelation sunk in. I broke into hysterics, exploding in an

97

orgasm of laughter that rose from some deep, secret place inside of me.

The next six weeks were a whirlwind. I kept finding myself floating into Mark's office under the guise of working on projects. Most of the time, I wasn't even sure how I got there. It was as if someone else had taken over my body and was speaking through me. I was a marionette, and an invisible guide was my puppet master pulling the strings.

I knew that I was hopelessly in love … and, for the first time in my life, consciously aware that I was completely out of control.

Mark was nothing like the men I was accustomed to being with. He was twelve years older than me and came from a family with a lot more money than I grew up with—a dyed-in-the-wool New Yorker who was incredibly outgoing.

He was successful. Established. And so stable.

It felt edgy, foreign, and exciting.

This was major unchartered territory. I didn't know how to navigate it.

I still hadn't broken things off with Steve. I couldn't seem to rip the Band-Aid off. A safety net, perhaps? Mark was divorced and worried about his kids. Both men were my work colleagues.

It was very, very messy.

I confided in a few close friends. They pointed out all the "red flags" and were concerned that I was being played and drawn into a rebound relationship.

I couldn't just leave my job, and it would take months to find a comparable position.

The only thing I could think to do was surrender. Allow it to happen and let the chips fall where they may.

And that's when the magic happened.

One night while Mark and I were on the phone talking about the future, I opened up about how raw and vulnerable I was. That the rational "had it all together" Lee had disintegrated. And that I had no idea what I was doing.

It was a leap of faith to stand before him, emotionally naked. Just me, stripped of my ego and all of my armor.

I fessed up: I did not know how to be in a healthy relationship. I didn't know if this would work. But I wanted to give it my all, with my whole heart. Could he help me?

We made promises to each other about how we wanted to be. We were honest about the rough road ahead and that there were no guarantees. But the one thing we could commit to, with certainty, was to keep the lines of communication open, and commit to working things through, always.

Thirteen years into our marriage, we are still guided by those promises. We live by our core motto, "Never boring, always evolving."

It gets better and better every day as I open to being more and more at ease with my life unfolding.

I am so grateful.

Reflection:

Have you ever purchased jewelry or something significant to represent your commitment to yourself? What did this gift bring you?

Where in your life are you living in or out of alignment? What can you do to increase your alignment?

Describe a time that you took a leap of faith and were vulnerable? What was the experience like and how did it change you to make that choice?

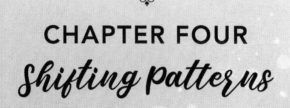

CHAPTER FOUR
Shifting Patterns

Befriending Anger

MARY JO RATHGEB

*W*hen I reached seven years old, I decided anger was bad. Since I wanted to be good, anger and I were sworn enemies. I felt tension and discomfort whenever anyone raised their voice or said mean things. Even when playing dolls with my sister, I always let her choose curvy Barbie, and I ended up with flat-chested Midge. I wanted Barbie too, but when my sister protested, I invariably deferred, swallowing my resentment and instead priding myself on playing nice.

As the "good girl," I believed not getting angry was admirable.

When I made that pact with my young self, I didn't realize all that I gave up by not allowing myself to connect with anger. I didn't know avoiding anger would impact my ability to stand in my power or speak up when needed, creating challenges in my relationships.

Fast-forward to adulthood, where my intention to be nice evolved into full-blown people-pleasing.

In my career, I was a model employee, got promoted, and managed a team. But I avoided conflict, which impacted my ability to lead effectively. I was once described as a doormat and sent to leadership training, where I discovered my long-honed strategy was actually self-defeating behavior, but I didn't know any other way to be.

In my personal life, whenever my partner and I fought, I would yell at him to stop being so angry. I blamed him for any fights we had. For a while, he believed me, too. He even sought help. After several months, he shocked me one day by saying that I was the hothead and that I was projecting my ire onto him.

What? Me? Angry? No way! What do you mean I am fr*@king angry? How dare you say that!

That night, I had a nightmare about my buried anger. In my dream, I descended a stone staircase into the depths of an ancient building. I was being summoned for the trial of a murder, and, in my heart, I knew I was guilty. I walked into the courtroom and sat on a backless wooden bench, dreading being there. As the judge looked at me and called my name, "MARY JO RATHGEB," I was whisked back to my ordinary life where I busily attended to mundane things, knowing I had to return to the subterranean courtroom and face my verdict.

In my dream, when I first returned to the cellar, the room appeared empty. With a slight shift of perception, I saw the space filled with people, and I sat on a bench along a stone wall.

Suddenly, Rage appeared from the dead in a puff of smoke. She was eight feet tall with wild red hair and a multicolored outfit resembling the Acid Queen from the movie, *Tommy*. She turned my way, pointed a boney finger at me, and screeched, "You! You killed me!"

I recoiled, knowing that she was coming for my jugular. I tried to warn everyone around me by shrieking that Rage would grab them by the throat, pin them to the wall, and choke them until they couldn't talk or breathe. I screamed. Then I woke up drenched in sweat.

I knew that I had to exhume my rage and shift my attitude towards it, which was easier said than done. I had buried anger so deeply that I didn't feel at all connected with it. Once I calmed down, I saw how my tendency to people-please impacted my ability, or inability, to express antagonism. I avoided conflict because I dreaded it. I wanted everyone to just get along, darn it! Instead of facing conflict, I gave my power away.

Once I *really* saw the issue, I couldn't unsee it. I noticed my irritability, my outbursts. Instead of rejecting my feelings or projecting blame on others, I got curious about what sparked my ire. I admit there were times I got frustrated or exasperated or, okay, yes, even downright indignant. I realized that being angry sometimes didn't make me a bad person. It made me human.

My experience of anger began to transform from being denied and demonized to honored and humanized.

With acceptance, I leaned in to better understand this fiery emotion. I started to put the pieces of the puzzle together and began dialoguing with anger, allowing it to express itself. I learned what triggered anger and how it sounded in my head. I even discovered anger had a sense of humor. Anger and I had a budding acquaintance.

Then, I came upon an emotional release technique called Regenerating Images in Memory (RIM). RIM helped me dive deeper into facing, understanding, and—eventually—befriending anger. During one RIM session, I saw anger as a gigantic beaker filled with pink acid, caustic and burning. I stepped into the liquid, allowed myself to feel the pain, and express my fury. The hurting stopped, and the liquid evaporated.

In another RIM session, I went to a childhood memory of a time I was mad at my mother. Since I hadn't ever expressed my feelings to her, they stayed frozen in my throat, rendering me speechless. As I paid attention to my throat, I noticed it was throbbing, and so I attended to that. As the sensations in my throat relaxed, my younger self expressed how she felt to my mom. This five-year-old version of me felt seen, heard, and valued. The experience shifted my feelings for my mother, and I saw that it was never too late to improve a relationship. Even though my mother died nearly thirty years ago, I felt closer to her than I had in decades.

In everyday life, I started to sit in the discomfort of indignation, allowing myself to be in it, letting it flow through my body and process as needed. I learned to face the ugliness or pain or however the displeasure presented. I learned the only way out is through. Afterward, I felt calm and peaceful in my body.

I am learning to trust anger, and, in turn, it teaches me its many facets. Turns out that this fiery emotion is not one-dimensional. It has layers and nuances. I created a new metaphor for this maligned energy, not as an acid that will burn me, but as a flame in a fire pit that, when properly contained, can be experienced as warming and purposeful.

Now, outrage alerts me when my boundaries have been crossed, or my values are in conflict. It lets me know when I am giving my power away. It highlights what is truly important to me. Antagonism provides motivation to get into action. It ignites passions. It also activates social interactions through sharing what I'm passionate about and creating healthy boundaries.

Befriending anger helped me be more direct in my interactions and has given me the ability to express myself more openly and honestly. My relationship with my partner is closer and more intimate than it has been in years. We now speak to each other about difficult or sensitive issues without necessarily getting combative or contentious. We allow each other to have our own perspective and acknowledge each perspective as valid, even if we don't agree with it. In fact, we often agree to disagree now.

A big insight for me was realizing that disagreeing and having conflicting views don't doom the relationship. Nor does it make me or him wrong or bad; it just makes us complex humans. I can have moments of annoyance, acknowledge it, ascertain its message, allow it to flow through me, and move from there. And I'm learning to be okay with my partner's displeasure too. It's a work in progress, but I have come a long way.

The journey to befriend anger began as a nightmare and a wake-up call. It has deepened into trusting and honoring the energy. By working with this emotion, instead of against it, I feel empowered and supported in so many unexpected ways. Changing my relationship to anger has transformed my relationship to myself and others. I would never have believed it possible until I started living it.

Reflection:

What is your relationship to anger and how is that impacting your relationships for better and for worse?

How would befriending anger transform your life?

What would be different for you if you implicitly trusted your anger?

Falling in Love

MARY MAGOUIRK

*I*t was mid-September 2022, and I stood in front of the bathroom mirror in my birthday suit, taking stock of what I saw looking back at me. "It's been a hell of a year so far," I muttered under a heavy sigh. "Eyes on the goal." My smooth face and colored hair belied my fifty-six years, six months, and twenty-two days. I loved that people who didn't know me often thought I was in my late thirties. They must have been picking up that I mentally felt like a thirty-something. But how my body felt was a whole other story.

Why was I standing in the mirror, naked, taking a mental picture of myself? A month and a half earlier, I was diagnosed with multiple sclerosis (MS). I had already had two overwhelmingly stressful months to prepare for the officialness of getting that diagnosis. I'd been through the short-term, fear-based panic of "Still single! Who's going to want me now? Who's going to be there to take care of me later on?" Once I got myself over that negative, panicky thinking, I'd come to the conclusion that I didn't want to go through the next chapter of my life uncoupled, as I was for much of the forty years preceding that rollercoaster in time.

A few days before this self-examination, I thought, "If I'm going to find my man, I need to really love myself. I think I love myself, but do I *really* love myself? Right now. As is." As much as I didn't want it to be the case, the deep down, tug-at-your-heart-and-soul answer was a resounding "No!"

The deep feeling I'd come to know intimately, of wondering if I would EVER find my man, was coupled with an echo that I had heard over and over from the chatterati, that "One must love themselves first. They must love their body."

I *thought* I always had loved my body. I talked to myself with kindness and was often surprised at hearing examples of other women picking themselves apart, saying mean things to themselves, and putting themselves down. Basically, the opposite of what I usually did. Occasionally, when passing by a mirror, I would say, "Hello, beautiful" to the reflection staring back at me. If I made a mistake or dropped an object, I'd tenderly exclaim, "That's brilliant, Mary!" with only the teensiest bit of sarcasm behind it. I loved myself long before I had ever heard of Louise Hay and her "mirror work."

I made a firm decision to fall in love with myself—my brain, my soul, my body—every inch! On the heels of a big weight loss and my new friend, the MS diagnosis, I looked in the mirror and made mental notes. With kindness, I evaluated what I saw. I cupped my hands under my sagging breasts, lifted them up to their once perky selves of my twenties and actual thirties, and felt their weight. I hadn't had kids. I hadn't nursed. I didn't have those perfectly acceptable reasons for the sag. A thought floated by, about standing in the buff for the first time with my potential love. I felt my shoulders roll forward at that thought. More questions began bubbling up. *How did the sag happen? Was it the fasting? Should I stop doing that? Was it the weight loss?*

I continued to size up the state of my breasts, then moved my gaze to the "still bigger than I'd like" tummy. The "still flabbier than I'd like" arms. I stood there, shifting from leg to leg, tilting my head the way my dog does, scanning the whole body, noticing the things I didn't love. I was kind, yet I still noticed it all.

I then made another decision—to love what I saw in the mirror. To really love myself, including the mind and the ethereal me housed by this body—that had breasts that didn't look like mine, a large tummy, cellulite, thinning hair. All of it. Love. Me.

I spent a few minutes each day on Project Love Me. I said things to myself in the mirror like, "Damn, you're beautiful! I love those luscious boobs. So soft and inviting. I love those soft, squishy parts. Just like a woman should be. Soft! And those curves, watch out, men!"

It didn't take long. Within a week, I DID absolutely love what I saw reflected back. I would cup my breasts and think about how it was awesome that they are soft, pliable, and more fun to play with than fake boobies that don't move. I loved the soft curviness of my body. I always loved myself, but now I also loved the body that "Myself" was in.

I began caressing my body. Not sexually, but sensually. I appreciated the act of looking at myself in the nude, with a soft, loving gaze, a growing smile. As I admired myself, I thought about how much I loved this body and its sexiness. Girlfriend, I even started to feel turned on by peering at myself and loving what I saw. I brought my natural sensuality back into my daily experience again, after it went missing some twenty years before. I was one with the beauty and sensuality and ALL those soft curves. Lots of curves. Lots of soft. I admired my breasts in a sexy bra, loving the soft, touchable cleavage it rendered.

While my brain was high on my own body, it told me that sleeping in the buff would amp up the sensuousness. And—it did! Ever the hopeless romantic from the time I could comprehend what that meant, I did what I do: surrounded myself with love songs and romance movies (yes, even the vilified Hallmark movies) for no other reason than I liked them. They're my jam.

You may be able to guess what happened next. All the soft

115

energy I was pouring into loving what I saw in the mirror, loving this body and the person IN the body, the curvy caresses, the love songs, and heady romance, had me thinking about being with a man. All the time. Thinking about passionate kisses and passionate lovemaking. Really FEELING him. I was fully present in the romantic lovemaking moments that played out in my mind.

And then, something truly remarkable happened. Without touching myself at all with my hands or with toys, I had a spectacular orgasm. The kind of orgasm I only had maybe twice before. Having been so awed by that, I continued the mental lovemaking and had multiple orgasms. For real. All without touching myself, other than gentle caresses of my hip curves and outer thighs. I was in a state of bliss.

Hallelujah! After decades of only being able to have orgasms from oral sex, I was over-the-moon ecstatic to learn that it IS possible for me to have an orgasm from (imagined) penetration alone, and multiple orgasms at that. I was able to duplicate this over and over again in the ensuing days. I came away from that experience with the full knowledge and understanding of how much loving ourselves and the actual body we are in plays a part in our sensual and sexual experiences. And how being *in love with ourselves* tops them all.

The power of visualization and "feelingization" (as author Arielle Ford calls it when one really gets into the feeling of having something) opened up a whole new world where it all worked together to create blissful magic! And those moments of blissful magic caused my mind to think about myself and a romantic relationship in a more empowered fashion. I began feeling like I didn't NEED a person in my life for the sake of having someone. "I got this. I can take my time. There is no hurry!" ran through my head.

All of this energetic shifting was felt outwardly as well. My "I've had the time of my life" man came back with majestic speed in a "magical manifestation" sort of way. And he loves all my parts.

Reflection:

If you were to stand before a mirror in your birthday suit, what messages would you give to yourself? Do these messages serve you?

How does self-love factor into your life?

Write down affirmations about your body that increase your self-love.

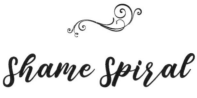

Shame Spiral

BONNIE SNYDER

*A*s their mother, I had hoped Leann and Michael would find partners who supported them in life. After a series of challenging relationships, Michael fell in love and married Carolyn. Their wedding vows were meaningful, filled with love and respect. When Michael's job took them across the country, new challenges presented themselves: smaller details of their life were unknown, and it felt like the fabric of our connection was unraveling.

Soon, Carolyn was late to Zoom calls. She remained quiet, yet I felt a tension in her demeanor. On one call, after not hearing from or seeing Carolyn for a bit, I cracked a joke conveying I was happy to see her. Carolyn misunderstood my attempt at humor and told me my comment hurt her feelings. I apologized, feeling terrible that my comment had caused such distress. Subsequent conversations were challenging, leaving me feeling misunderstood and like the "bad guy."

When Michael said they were coming for a visit, I was glad, as was Leeann and her family, who lived nearby. I was anxious about the visit. In addition to our difficult conversations, when they last visited, I seemed to fall short of creating a comfortable experience as I like to do for my guests. It felt like I couldn't say or do anything right.

After they arrived, the tension felt like a heavy winter blanket. Carolyn barely spoke. But as the evening went on, the chill lifted. Everyone started to relax, laugh, and converse more easily.

The next day Leeann, Michael, and I talked about taking a family picture. No pressure—or so I thought! I suggested we coordinate colors around the clothing Carolyn and Michael had with them. I could never have anticipated a simple request for a family photo would result in a year of shame, angst, and family disruption.

Later, as Michael and I were talking, Carolyn walked into the room. I asked if those were the blue pants Michael suggested she wear for the picture. To my surprise, Carolyn interjected in an angry voice, explaining that she resented what I had done five years earlier when we had taken family pictures. She recalled how I told her she should wear a different top or find anything different than what she was going to wear. What? I would never tell someone to do anything like that. But this is how she remembered the interaction.

I was frozen in shock. Her words were like a punch in the stomach. I didn't know what to say. I was hurt and stung by her words. My heart ached. The only thing I knew to say right then was it was hard for me to process what was said when I was spoken to unkindly. Carolyn walked out of the house. I followed to attempt to discuss, but she didn't want to talk.

My husband thought it best to get some distance, and we left to go out to dinner. I fell apart, shedding a waterfall of tears. I felt confusion and shame that my son's wife felt that way. I had no idea she had been holding on to these feelings. My husband was angry at how Carolyn spoke disrespectfully to me. He reassured me what we both heard was untrue.

When we arrived home, Michael asked if the three of us could talk. As we sat down, Carolyn started a litany of painful places for her and how I had contributed to this pain over the last few years.

Carolyn thought I was controlling when I asked the family to coordinate colors for the family picture. She thought gifts and conversations around different ideas for self-development, which she expressed an interest in, were offered to make her a better person for her husband. These ideas are what my "work" is about for me and my clients. I share them with everyone.

Carolyn's ending comment was how I "never thought about how what I said affected others."

I was devastated and felt like I had been burned. For much of my life, I've worried what I said or did might hurt the other person. I went to bed sobbing. I knew friends, clients, and even strangers who viewed me as a safe person to talk to, understanding and non-judgmental of their challenges. I couldn't reconcile what had happened. A cloak of shame smothered me. For the remainder of the visit, Carolyn didn't speak to me.

That started the year of silence.

I cried, processed, and used my toolbox of strategies to handle my pain and emotional distress. Right from the start, as much as I hated it, I knew I needed to learn from the experience. The first was to look at my sensitivity around patterns of hurt and shame. I felt like I had been cut open and stabbed in the heart, devastated by shame that, throughout my life, had been an unwelcome companion.

Then came the anger. Using anger against myself was an automatic response, a maladaptive coping strategy, which may be attributed to my high sensitivity. I stayed caught in a continuous loop of self-criticism, shame, and anger.

I had been having trouble with my back, and it had gotten worse. As my holistic practitioner worked on my physical body, he found repressed anger. It was like I had physically taken a fall. My emotions had literally twisted my spine and caused a "fall" from my authentic self. 121

In my family, we'd always been able to work through challenging relationships, including divorces. My heart ached that I couldn't "fix" this problem. There was a large hole in the fabric of our family that might never be stitched together.

I knew that Carolyn had been subject to traumatic experiences, and I felt compassion for her. At one point, I was angry with myself for being so compassionate. I knew how important it was for me to completely transform my inner shame, frustration, and anger in appropriate ways. Most painful was my concern for Michael and his pain of being in the middle between two people he loved.

A year later, before an upcoming visit, Carolyn emailed me and suggested a joint therapy session. I agreed. I had seen many women with adult children stuff their feelings down to avoid conflict with their children's spouses. Even if the relationship was strained, they would keep quiet to avoid being cut off from their children or grandchildren. Despite my trepidation, I knew I had to follow through and see where this took us.

During the first session, Carolyn talked about how difficult she found our relationship. A hopeless feeling settled in, and my stomach was in knots. After more inner work and focusing on forgiveness, I woke before our second session clear about what I needed to say. I felt my heart open up to Carolyn. It was important not to continue the energy of separation and to have the courage to lean into my sensitivity about others' judgment toward me.

The second session did not go well until the last ten minutes when Carolyn burst into tears and said she didn't want to be thought of as a "disrespectful and unkind person."

Surprised by her words, I said, "I don't think of you that way. I just felt that I had been spoken to disrespectfully and unkindly in two conversations."

Like glass shattering, there was a shift. Carolyn apologized for taking a year holding on to her feelings, didn't want to come between Michael and me, and knew how much I cared for both of them. It was a miracle! Despite my ability to support others with shame in my coaching practice, this painful year taught me much. It allowed me to stop repressing my feelings, release my own shame, to stand up for myself in a more assertive way, and to stop turning against myself. I reclaimed parts of myself that for years have kept me from being my authentic self and to lean into, own, and honor myself and my sensitivity more fully.

Reflection:

Have you ever had a conflict with a family member that left you feeling badly? How did you resolve the issue? What would you do differently?

In what ways do you exercise your assertiveness? What messages do you receive when you do so? Are these messages helpful?

Describe the tools you use to navigate difficult or challenging situations.

Wow

CRYSTAL COCKERHAM

*W*ow, an entire world just opened up. It felt surreal and unbelievable, as if I were living in my imagination. I had heard of this experience in movies and on television shows, and I had read about it in books, but I had never made the connection that being an empath was a real thing.

"Crystal, you are an empath!"

The news came as a shock. I was temporarily paralyzed, frozen in time. In all honesty, I cannot for the life of me remember what the conversation was before those words made it to my ears.

What I do remember as I came to terms with the reality of being an empath, was something my college English professor had said about there being no original ideas. That everything here on earth was cocreated with divine grace. It was a light bulb moment: of course, having empathic abilities was a real thing! Where else had those writers for television, movies, and books found their ideas?

Discovering, acknowledging, and accepting that I am an empath brought a seismic life shift. It came early on in my journey as a lightworker and opened the door to an entire library of lessons. Only now, as I sit to recollect this part of my story, do I see the accelerated speed in which this aspect of my journey was on. As I have mentioned in previous writings, once the divine knew it had my attention, the first two years were full of turbo-speed transformations and *a-ha* moments!

During those first two years, as I woke up from the deep slumber of the fears and false masks I had been hiding under, my eyes opened to the world of energy healing with essential oils, crystals, and coaching. I had come home to myself in the soul-quenching circle of sacred ceremony and the divine feminine energies. In hindsight, I recognize that each one was a keystone in the foundation of my spiritual journey with embracing my empathic gifts as the fourth.

I had a lot to learn about what it meant to be an empath; it was unknown territory for me. And it was vital to my health, my mental and emotional well-being, and my spiritual maturity that I do so.

This learning did not happen overnight, and it wasn't easy. The more I felt into it and worked with this part of me, the easier it became and the more of me—the real me—I met.

One of my first tasks was to discern my feelings from other people's. Discerning my feelings from others was the most difficult part of this process. Why? Because I had developed coping mechanisms as a child that were the only way I knew then and, like any wounded part of myself, I had to unravel it—break it down—and examine each part so I could learn the truth and understand it in order live holistically as an empath.

During this accelerated part of my awakening, I audited every aspect of my life. I learned to trust myself, and to trust in what I believed and what I wanted. I kept saying that I couldn't wait to meet myself.

Embracing the fact that I was an empath was the last big reveal the divine had for me. Accepting this aspect of myself finally gave me the stability I needed to begin fully embodying the real me and breaking free from the falsities I had been living under.

I could no longer allow my true self to hide.

You see, I had been feeling everyone else's feelings my entire life but had no idea! What's worse was, growing up, my feelings weren't validated unless it was in a negative way, so I had decades' worth of un-conditioning to do as well. I know that many readers are going to know exactly what I am talking about. If you are one of them, I say to you, "Your feelings are real; they are true for you. It doesn't matter if anyone else believes you or not. It only matters that you know, that you believe."

As I practiced this discernment, I noticed something BIG: every time I found myself feeling something that wasn't mine, I felt sick to my stomach. My body helped me discern my feelings from someone else's through physical cues. Guess what? I had had all sorts of tummy issues my entire life!

Every time I felt feelings that I didn't think were mine, I energetically cleared them using a variety of tools, such as meditation, visualization, essential oils, crystals, receive energy work, etc. Then I would call in Archangel Michael and envision an energetic field of protection. Do you know what happened? I became more confident and expedient with my discernment, and I experienced a lot less tummy trouble!

Do I tune into other people's feelings on purpose? No. No way! I have enough of my own feelings, thank you very much. If someone else's feelings show up for me during a client session, I know it is a cue for me to inquire about them. If it is during some other form of interaction, I know it is far more a signal for me— guidance, if you will—as to how I should or shouldn't engage with a particular person for mine and their highest and greatest good. In this way, I have embraced being an empath as a gift. A superpower even.

129

You might be thinking that this is the end of my story, of my life shift. It isn't. This was just the beginning for me to lean into this new inner navigation system.

What I learned for myself as an empath was that it didn't begin or end with feeling other people's feelings. It was simply part of it. Also, part of being an empath was being highly in tune with my intuition and being able to feel the energy of a space or situation, down to if a food or event is good for me or not.

In my experience of supporting and guiding others, in addition to my own path of learning, I realized that the more intuitive a person is, the more sensitive, or empathic, they become. For me, I learned to hone my empathic gifts before I worked on strengthening my intuition. However, the more I worked on mastering my empathic senses, the more aware and open I became intuitively. The more I learned about my intuitive nature, the more I realized it, too, had been with me all along.

In fact, I found myself remembering flashes from childhood such as: making my own "perfume" with the wild roses I picked from the fence line of the farmer's field where I had my fort, or when I was in kindergarten, knowing there was something wrong with my dad when he called even though he didn't tell me. (He was hurt badly at work as a result of a machine malfunctioning. He ended up having surgery and was hospitalized for weeks.)

In reflecting upon the memories that surfaced, I learned how my intuitive and empathic abilities had been an innate part of my very being. Yet, I didn't have anyone to teach me while I was young. It was my task as an awakened woman to dive into my past and retrieve what I needed so that I could teach myself how to tap into and wield the innate gifts I truly believe we are all born with so that I could then better help others do the same.

A good handful of years later, I went and visited my great-aunt in the hospital. I felt the nudge to ask her about intuition and, specifically, tea leaf reading. Even now, thinking about this experience, I tear up. Apparently, the gifts were powerful in that branch of my family tree, as evidenced by the fact that my great-grandmother, her mother, and sister could predict a family birth within minutes of the actual time recorded! My Mimmi passed away when I was in high school and my aunt not long after that conversation. I feel their presence sometimes. I hear their voices or a voice that feels like the voice of my ancestors. They wait patiently at each gateway. They are always there guiding me, like when I entered that next embodiment by initiating into the divine feminine and again when I entered into my queendom, deepening my inner work, and when leading ceremony for myself and others.

Now, my eyes are wide open. I am not afraid to feel. To be. What I discovered is this: there is magic in each and every moment. When you are open and fully present in the now, time practically stands still. It is in this moment you can see, feel, hear, taste, and touch everything while still fully being your sovereign self.

Wow.

Reflection:

What gifts have you received from your family?

How do you notice and appreciate the magic of everyday moments?

Where in your body does your intuition show up? What happens when you listen to your intuitive hits? What happens when you don't?

Learning to Dance with the Universe

LISA HROMADA

I felt my stomach tighten and my breathing become shallow as I prepared to enter the room. The hallway was eerily quiet. I wondered if anyone would show up. I'd invited a few friends to sit in the audience in hopes that their presence would soothe my uneasiness, but I didn't know if they'd show. I felt an all-too-familiar sting of being alone, unsupported, and not important enough. I was about to speak in front of a live audience for the very first time.

"This is no big deal," I silently tried to convince myself. "You can do this."

I watched my mom, one of my only solid supporters in my life, pace toward the back of the venue hall. She was pushing a stroller that my twenty-month-old daughter was napping in, taking care of her so that I could share the spiritual teachings that she had handed down to me. Part of me was excited to share my parents' supernatural experiences, to tell people how my dad channeled messages from the spirit world. And part of me was terrified. I grew up with a fear of the spotlight. I lacked self-confidence, and

135

as an empathic, sensitive introvert, I often felt that no one wanted to hear what I had to say. Nonetheless, I knew that I was meant to share these spiritual teachings and couldn't let my fear stop me.

I walked into the room, trying not to let my nervousness show as I shuffled my papers in my hands. I made my way up to the podium and looked out at the small gathering of people. Anxiously, I began.

"Imagine an evening like any other. Only this evening, your spouse comes home and says, 'After putting the kids to bed tonight, I need you to sit next to me and take notes as souls speak through me.'"

As I stood in front of the audience, I could feel my heart beating faster and faster. The sound of it was like a thousand drums pounding in my ears, and the tension building up inside began to overwhelm me.

Still, I did my best to continue speaking. "It was September twenty-first, nineteen-eighty-one, when this happened between my parents. My father … came home from work … and …" If my shaky, sweaty hands or quivering voice didn't reveal my intense fear of being *seen* for what felt like the first time in my life, then this moment certainly did. I froze. Mid-sentence. My mind was empty of all the words I had practiced for months.

"I'm sorry. I have to stop," I confessed. Hiding my humiliation and lack of poise and perfection, I closed my eyes and took a deep breath. In and out, in and out. And as I did, I felt a presence of calm fill me. I opened my eyes.

"Let me start again."

This moment of recentering was only the first of many life shifts I would have as I openly accepted my role in sharing these spiritual teachings. It would also be the first of the many divine (and often uncomfortable) nudges by the Universe for me to peel away the layers of fears and limiting beliefs that, over the years, had stifled my confidence and kept me feeling small in my life. Ironically, the path that I was being called to take at the age of thirty-eight would not only be paved with a purpose to share spirit-led messages of love, beauty, and personal empowerment. It would also be paved with personal challenges, disappointments, and triumphs that would gradually reveal a potential in me I didn't even know existed. It was as though the Universe placed me on a path to learn and fully live out what I was ultimately meant to share and teach others—that although challenges are inevitable, there is infinite potential within each to experience joy, purpose, and radical self-acceptance. Love is at the seed of it all.

This first speaking event was the start of a profound shift in my life. One in which I would be required to fully step out of my comfort zone and onto a path to find my voice, fully accept my imperfections, and fulfill a purpose that I innately knew, even as a child, that I was destined for. Years before I stepped onto that stage, I remember listening to a cassette tape of an astrology reading that my parents had done for me when I was two years old, in which it was said that I would be "a speaker for God." It would take three decades to begin learning what that meant.

Here's the funny thing about life. You can have a plan, purpose, and destiny, but that doesn't mean the journey will be smooth. It often isn't. There will be hurdles to jump and mountains to climb. Yet, in hindsight, I can see how every challenge, dead-end, and detour along my path served a purpose to awaken me to a higher potential dormant inside.

Answering the initial soul whispers that told me to share the channeled sessions set me on a path to healing the limitations I placed on myself and to following a career path that would be both empowering for me as well as those I served. As Joseph Campbell notably said, "We must let go of the life we have planned, so as to accept the one that is waiting for us."

137

By trusting in an uncertain path, meeting fears, stretching outside my comfort zone, and following the work that called to my heart, I experienced more and more small, yet significant life shifts. As I began my career, empowering women on their spiritual and life journeys, I too was on a similar journey. I began to question deep-seated limiting beliefs around self-worth and self-acceptance. I sought programs on mindset and ritually implemented other spiritual practices in order to gain the confidence I needed to not only fulfill my purpose through this work but also to feel happier and more in control of my life. And I did.

In questioning my limiting beliefs, I began to heal them. The more I healed them, the more confident I became. And the more confident I became, the more courage I had to share the wisdom that was placed in my heart. The more courageous I was, the more the Universe would place the right people, the right resources, the right mentors, and the right opportunities along my path. I was learning what it is to dance with the Universe. To trust in the flow and process of being and becoming who and what I'm meant to be.

I discovered that every challenge, success, and step along an uncertain path would lead me to experience what happens when we make the choice to see life through a new set of eyes. To see the possibilities beyond the fears and the potential beyond the limiting beliefs. Although it felt uncomfortable at times, I knew that I was not just meant to be a speaker or a writer, but to be an uplifter and a keeper of the light so that others may find it. As I continued to follow my heart and moved beyond my fears, I realized a destiny that was available to me all along. And with every step I took, the Universe never left my side. Doors opened that I didn't know were there, and people came into my life to support and guide me along the way.

I experienced a shift from fear to love, resistance to peace, limitations to possibilities, and from problems to solutions. I've realized that every challenge along the way has awakened me to what's truly possible. With courage, trust, patience, and perseverance, I'm continually reassured that, just as the souls and Wise Ones shared in those channeled sessions, everything I need is here with me now – the wisdom, love, and guidance, all divinely seeded in me.

Life works in unexpected ways. It often leads you toward paths that push your boundaries, pull you out of the comfort of your shell, and call you to climb higher than you believe is possible. It's been my truth in recent years that there is infinite potential to create a meaningful, uplifting, and fulfilling life of purpose. I've learned not to ignore that calling inside and that part that says, "Maybe it's possible." Just maybe I am here to create something powerful.

Reflection:

Where might you be letting fear hold you back from giving your gifts?

What do you need to *do* or how do you need to *be* to create more joy in your life?

What limiting beliefs do you need to change to become the person you're being called to become?

CHAPTER FIVE
Shifting Self-Realization

My Near-Death Experience

MARIA BURKE, RN

*F*or weeks, I had a vivid and recurring dream where I saw a car hydroplane and spin out of control. I thought it was a premonition that someone close to me was going to be in a car accident. All my family and friends were sick of me asking the same question: are you wearing your safety belt? If their response was no, I shared my dream and begged them to please wear their safety belt.

One Sunday morning, it rained in a way that reminded me of Ireland. There, we have an expression describing heavy rain: lashing rain. I left home and drove into Boston, the pelting rain so heavy I could barely see. I had just passed Braintree when suddenly my car hydroplaned, and I lost control. My car slammed twice into the barrier on the left-hand side before launching into a spin, my car careening across five lanes of traffic before coming to a stop in the left lane facing oncoming traffic.

While this unfolded, it felt familiar; I had experienced this accident in my dream. Unafraid, I bent my head and took my hands off the steering wheel. I felt a warm, intense wave of love that started at my toes and spread through my body before the energy exited through my head. I felt the Blessed Mother Mary behind me, her

145

arms outstretched as if she wanted to hug me. I felt and saw this blinding white light—I had never seen anything so bright. The light engulfed me, and I felt myself surrounded by love and light. Time stood still; I felt weightless, like I was floating.

At this time, my children were exceedingly young, and their faces flashed before me. Even though I wanted to keep going into the light, I begged our Blessed Mother to please not take me as I wanted to be there for my children.

The next thing I knew, I heard someone tapping at the driver's side window. A doctor who practiced at Brigham and Women's Hospital had pulled over and parked in front of my car in the fast lane in case another car hit my car. I stared straight ahead, in a total daze, unsure of where I was.

He said, "Don't move. I don't want you to injure yourself further." He stayed with me until the rescue team arrived, and I never got an opportunity to thank him, a godsend during a scary time.

A female state trooper arrived first and, after reassuring me that an ambulance was on its way, parked her cruiser in front of the doctor's car. She redirected traffic, which was challenging due to the rain and limited visibility.

The EMTs arrived and immediately put a neck brace on me while I was still in the car. They asked, "Do you have any pain or shortness of breath?"

"No," I said.

"Can you feel your legs?"

I suddenly realized that I couldn't.

The firefighters cut me out of the car and held their helmets over me as shelter from the rain while they transferred me on a stretcher to the ambulance, which sped its way to nearby Quincy Hospital. Suddenly, I was swarmed by a huge team of doctors and nurses. I heard the EMT give a report, and I felt the concern in his voice as he shared that my car was totaled. At the time, I drove a Volvo, which I feel was a contributing factor to my survival.

In the hospital, I had every test imaginable. The doctor was

146

amazed that I was okay (feeling returned to my legs, thankfully) and discharged me that very same day! I had no idea that after this event, my whole life would change.

At the time of the accident, I worked in South Boston as a hairdresser. I loved being a hairdresser and had also worked as a stylist in London before opening my own salon in Ireland.

After the accident, I felt totally changed. I still felt intense love for my profession, but being a hairdresser no longer fulfilled me. I had not told anyone about my experience, and even though I tried to rationalize my feelings away, I could not even explain it to myself. I became fascinated with any books or materials related to near-death experiences. I knew this had happened to me for a reason; I just had to figure out why.

I had always wanted to go to college. Unfortunately, this was not an option for me in Ireland. After my accident, on a whim, I decided to apply to nursing school at Labouré College. To my surprise, I was interviewed, took the entrance exam, and was admitted into their nursing program that very day!

After I graduated, my first position was at Boston Medical. During this time, I took care of a lot of patients. One particular patient had AIDS. He was terrified of dying. I shared my near-death experience with him; he said it brought him comfort. Sadly, one night while I worked the night shift, he suddenly declined and ultimately passed away.

This event changed my nursing journey. Up until then, I had not shared my near-death experience with anyone. I realized that my story could be a gift because many people are terrified of dying. I pivoted to become a hospice nurse and started my own home health care company. It is such an honor and privilege to be able to help our patients pass away in their own homes while at the same time providing comfort to their families.

During the dying process, the soul travels from this world to the next. I have been at the bedside of many of our patients when they have transitioned. Some patients have seen children surrounding their beds. Some semi-lucid patients talked about travel or said they were preparing to go on a trip. Some patients have told me that their parents were there to take them home. Some have seen angels while in a semiconscious state and would smile or appear to be conversing with someone. I share this because I don't want you to be afraid if your loved one tells you that they saw or had a conversation with a loved one who has passed.

I have felt the energy shift at the moment of passing, and I believe that anyone in the room receives a special blessing. I realized that death is just a new beginning and a natural part of living. As Saint Michael said, "Love is the most important thing."

Reflection:

What did you learn from a difficult experience and how did that knowledge transform your life?

Have you or a loved one ever had a near-death experience? Describe what it was like. What was the gift that came from having had this experience?

In what ways has your life's journey been non-traditional? How has this difference guided you to new opportunities?

Discovering the Power Within

CAMY DE MARIO

I grew up a child of privilege in Milan, Italy, with parents and a brother. My mom took her own life when my brother and I were teenagers. Our dad counterbalanced for our loss by providing beautiful homes and sumptuous vacations. As a restaurateur, he poured himself into his work. Being generous with money seemed to be his way of showing love, compensation for him not being overly present, physically or emotionally, in our lives. I knew I could always count on him. How lovely to never worry about money or bills! He never denied me, even when I told him that I wanted to move my family to Florida and asked him for financial support.

Within six months, my then-husband and I moved our family to Palm Beach, Florida, settling on a new continent and in a new home. We also bought a business—all while raising our young daughter, three and a half years old, and son, one and a half. My marriage crumbled within five years as my husband, who desperately missed Italy, had a difficult time adjusting to our new way of life.

My husband returned to Italy with our children, leaving me in Florida with the business. I saw my life, ambitions, and dreams

151

crash before me. I had thought money and this new venture would make us happy, but it didn't. I lost everything financially, and I felt completely broken emotionally.

I tried to keep myself above water, scrambled to sell the business, and move back to Italy. I missed my children horribly, and it wasn't easy to communicate with my ex-husband, so I prayed a lot for a miracle to happen to take me out of that mess. As usual, I expected outside sources to fix my problems instead of counting on my own resilience and strength. I stayed in Palm Beach and traveled back and forth to Italy to see my children, while still running a business that slowly failed. Eventually, I was forced to close it for good.

Then, unexpectedly, Bobby walked into my life. He came in as a tornado, bringing excitement, devotion, and so much love. I realized he was my mirror, a man who also lived a privileged life, and understood my needs. We connected immediately, although I waited a year before saying "yes" to his marriage proposal (we've been married twenty-three years!). We traveled extensively, and he showed me beautiful places that I always wanted to visit. We lived the life of millionaires, on a trust fund, between Palm Beach, the Bahamas, Aspen, and California. Our home base was in Southern California, and our youngest children, twins, attended middle school in an affluent area near Malibu.

We lived a high life until one day when we learned that our trust fund was depleted. We lost everything. Our world crashed down in a split second, and we were forced to face a brutal reality.

We saw no other way but to move our children and our two pets into a shabby Motel 6 and rely on some support from a few friends, trying to figure out how to face the future. At that moment, it felt like lightning struck me. My husband fell apart, and I realized that I was the "heart" of our family and felt the responsibility to keep the family together.

Despite feeling terrified, I became determined to change our circumstances, focusing not only on regaining financial stability, but also growing spiritually and emotionally. Despite the challenges, the Universe called me to trust myself, and to rely on the power of prayers.

I demonstrated to my family that our future could be brighter because of our perseverance to break through any challenges. I wanted to become a better person, change my karma, and heal my relationship with money. I listened to that inner voice, accepting every divine message from the Universe as my only real guidance.

Gratitude became an essential part of my daily life, and I saw miracles because of my humility to say "thank you" even when things were not perfect. The fact that my family remained intact was an opportunity to celebrate and receive blessings.

At that time in my life, I had a deep spiritual awakening. As much as life was difficult and living in a Motel 6 with young children is not what anyone would wish for, I had the opportunity to meet interesting people, a few of them going through a similar experience. What struck me the most was that these folks had a complete trust that their circumstances would turn around. I sat with them, shared my fears, and they found ways to encourage me. They had wisdom, and I witnessed their victories. Their triumphs helped me to awaken to a new world of possibilities.

I also rediscovered talents that I had suppressed. I found the time and inspiration to start a new career as a children's book author and illustrator. I accepted several freelance positions as an illustrator that brought in some funds and helped with some bills. After a year of uncertainty, we moved into a new home back in Florida.

Sometimes, history repeats itself, which proved true for me. Six months ago, we were displaced from the home we'd rented for six years. I sat in disbelief that this had happened again; the fears of being displaced (I don't like to use the term "homeless") caught me abruptly, so that, for a while, I didn't have the chance to bring myself back to that state of calm and trust—until someone reminded me of my purpose. I am here to teach and guide everyone

153

that crosses my path. My life is not anymore about "having" but "being." Being a notable example of self-worth, resilience, and determination. Again, I trusted the Universe to continue blessing me through my work and service to others.

Life has a different meaning now, and I enjoy taking each day at a time. While all of my children have grown up into wonderful and responsible human beings, I spend every day trying to leave an impact on everyone that I come across. I love sharing my artistic talents and ensuring that everyone understands the importance of believing in themselves when facing challenges. When it comes to art, holding a paintbrush can be a way to feel free to explore any possibilities. A blank canvas can be the tool to step into a world of manifestation.

I now really enjoy sitting outside our new home while the birds are singing, and I'm surrounded just by nature; my heart radiates with joy. I have finally learned to be happy with just the simple things.

Reflection:

How have you clung to messages of value and worth that stemmed from your childhood? Do these beliefs serve you? What would you change?

Compile a list of good things that came from adversity. Reflect on these gifts.

Where does shame show up for you? What is its origin? Does it serve you or can it be transmuted into something that does serve you?

The Best Thing You Can Be Is Yourself

NANCY OKEEFE

I was very fortunate to grow up in a new, suburban neighborhood of nearly identical ranch houses, all with pretty yards and slightly different paint schemes that made each house look unique. Everyone moved into the neighborhood at the same time, and all the families had kids the same age. It was so easy to feel included and make friends. All I had to do was go out in my front yard to find girls jumping rope or roller skating and boys playing catch or dodgeball in the street. A short bike ride away was a park with swings, a giant slide, a merry-go-round, a baseball field, and plenty of kids. In the winter, on any school snow day, we had the best sledding hill right at the top of my street. Everyone was my friend, some closer than others, but we all hung out together like one big friend group, being ourselves and having the best time. I belonged simply because I lived there, in that little neighborhood in New Jersey.

There were two schools all the kids in my neighborhood went to: Public School 14 and St. Andrews. We all walked to and from school together and played together after school. It didn't matter which school you went to; they were right next to each other. But at twelve years old, like everyone else, I had to leave my neighborhood school for junior high in another part of town. My friends disappeared into other homerooms and classes, and I was faced with making all new school friends. I wasn't too worried. I had tons of friends and never doubted my ability to make more.

I quickly learned that the unconditional acceptance I enjoyed in my neighborhood also disappeared with my neighborhood friends. Friendship cliques formed quickly, and I was left struggling to find my new posse. Being accepted in school became as important as math and history. To make matters worse, a few months into the school year, just when I was just settling in, my father changed jobs, and we moved to rural Maryland. That was now our home.

Our new house was much bigger than the three-bedroom ranch we used to live in. The weather was warmer, and there was more country and less city. There were a few kids on our street, but I had to go looking for them, or worse, knock on their front doors and talk to their moms to find someone to hang out with. I started another new school. It was scary, and everything was a bit different.

As it turned out, this time it was much harder to make new friends. It was almost the middle of the school year and friendships had already been formed. In this new school, we changed classrooms constantly, with no time to socialize in between. It was a chaotic rush to get to my next class before the late bell rang. The only people to talk to were the kids on either side of me during class. You could sneak in a word or two when the teacher wasn't looking, but it was hard to make friends that way.

I wasn't accepted or welcomed into any group. I looked different. My accent was different. My clothes were different, and as the new kid, I got teased a lot. I suppose I've always been a bit different, a rebel of sorts. The status quo didn't stick with me. My thought process is different. I'm curious and questioning. I don't accept things at face value, and sometimes I see possibilities that others don't. I've always known that, but it never made a difference in my ability to make friends before. I felt lost and alone. I spent a lot of time in my new bedroom after school, longing for a friend and wondering what I could do to fit in.

Little by little, I started changing myself to survive. A well-timed growth spurt led to my mother taking me shopping for new school clothes. I nagged her to let me get clothes like the popular girls wore. It was a battle, but she finally gave in and let me get one or two outfits I wanted. These clothes weren't like anything I would have ever picked for myself before but were necessary to fit in. I changed my hair by teasing it up and choking on a cloud of hair spray. I started reading teen magazines and hanging out in the girls' bathroom, putting on makeup in between classes so my mother wouldn't see it. The more I conformed, the more I was accepted. I barely recognized myself in the mirror, but I finally fit in and made friends.

It wasn't any different in high school. I learned that conforming was the key to being popular. Conforming and being a little daring. A little shock value got you a few cool points. I had always been adventurous, so the daring part was easy, but the stakes got higher in high school. Eventually, my makeup routines in the girls' bathroom turned into smoke breaks and walking home from school with my new friends included drinking beer and hanging with boys.

By the end of high school, I was a master at fitting in, but I barely recognized myself. I had tons of friends in several groups. I was included and confident again. When I went off to look for work, getting hired meant changing myself again. The rules for acceptance at work and getting ahead required dressing for success, acting a certain way, and knowing when to speak and when not to. I did what was expected and fell into a very successful pattern. I advanced at work and received raises, promotions, and awards. I was successful at fitting in and being what someone wanted right up through my first marriage and my first baby. I had a storybook life, exactly the life you would have expected a kid who grew up in a perfect neighborhood of perfect families to have.

But one day, my perfect life didn't feel like my life anymore. It wasn't a dramatic moment. Nothing earth-shattering happened, but suddenly I realized I had become so good at conforming to everyone else's picture of success that, except for being a mother, there was nothing else in my life that I wanted. I felt lost and alone again. Not because there weren't people around me and not because I didn't feel loved and successful, but because I did. I had lost myself and forgotten what made me feel alive.

I wanted to be free to be myself again and do whatever I wanted to do whenever I wanted to do it. It was like someone switched on a light, and I could see the parts of myself that had been hiding in the dark for so long. I realized that conforming to what others think you should do and who you should be had taken its toll on me. It's exhausting to be something you are not.

My life changed dramatically in that one quiet moment. I had a newfound clarity about who I was and what I wanted. I began to politely say, "No, thank you" to things that I didn't want to do and people I didn't want to be with. I felt free, joyful, unapologetic, and comfortable in my own skin for the first time in a long time. Overnight, I had more interests and hobbies, with the energy to pursue them. I started painting and crafting. I loved flowers and art. I tried every medium I could. I had limitless creativity that I hadn't experienced before. I took classes on art and flower arrangement and met others who shared my interests. I felt real, and life was effortless. I felt like a kid again.

The moment I decided to be myself and follow my heart no matter what anyone else thought reshaped the rest of my life, and I achieved things personally and professionally that I never dreamed possible: author, speaker, entrepreneur, leader, and coach.

Be different. Be yourself. That's what attracts the right people

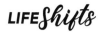

and experiences into the life you are meant to live; a rich life full of ease, flow, happiness, and friends that love you for who you are.

Reflection:

Are there places in your life where you're trying to fit in?
Why is it important to fit in?

How do you embrace and value your differences?

What "rules" are meant to be broken? What will it mean
for you if you chose to break them?

Coming Full Circle from Loss to Joy

AMY LINDNER-LESSER

*M*exico. Its ancient mysteries and brilliant colors first attracted me at twelve when my family spent our summer vacation there. It called me back at thirteen for an immersive exchange program. During college, my parents and I explored more of Mexico. And when I struggled to conceive, my late husband Steve and I adopted our daughters, Nina and Maya, from Mexico, which required that we live there for five magical weeks each time.

When our older daughter, Nina, was two, we hosted a Mexican exchange student. Two years later, when we adopted Maya, we went to Chihuahua to finish the process. Our exchange student's family opened their home to us during our extended stay.

Mexico has always held a special place in my heart. Once Maya told me that I was more Mexican than she was, and she was born there! The last time I visited Mexico was when Maya, now nearly thirty-five, was a toddler.

In December 2020, I hosted a retreat at my former inn for a woman who is a sensei, a shaman. She leads shamanic journeying using no drugs or alcohol. I took part in the retreat.

On my journey, I sat in a town square someplace in Mexico. I couldn't identify the town, but it felt familiar. I told the other participants that my journey had been a great dream, but going back to Mexico was probably not going to happen. I had commitments to my family, my business, and my friends.

Two weeks later, the inn's doorbell rang.

It was a realtor who said, "I have people who are interested in purchasing your inn."

I said, "I love what I'm doing. I love my guests." And then the voice in the back of my head reminded me that "every business is for sale if the price is right." I told the realtor to bring his buyers. I'd talk to them, show them around, listen to any offers, and then decide what to do.

Right after Christmas, they came, looked, made an offer, and within a few days of negotiating, I accepted. Three months later, I packed up more than twenty-five years of possessions—mine, my parents', and my children's leftovers from when they moved out. I found a house and moved to another state—all in six weeks.

Retired life was not for me, so I attended a retreat where I decided that I would provide coaching and consulting services for innkeepers to help them rediscover the joy of their chosen career. That's how INNtrospection was born.

A year later, I realized that working with innkeepers, while still a passion of mine, was not necessarily a priority of theirs. So, I took the gifts from my BFF of forty-four years' August 2022 death and began offering loss, grief, and life transition coaching.

The first week of March can be triggering for me as my mother passed away on March 4, and March 5 was Steve's birthday. So, when I received an invitation to attend a retreat in Mexico happening during that time, I knew I had to attend. I saw it as a way to complete a circle that started when I was twelve.

When it looked like retreat registrations were slow and the event happening iffy, I kept saying, "I'm going to be in Mexico for this week. I know it's going to happen because the Universe wants it to happen for me." And it did!

The day before I left for Mexico, I looked out my window and saw a male and a female cardinal hanging out for a long time in a tree in my backyard. It is said that cardinals represent loved ones who have passed. I believe that they were Steve, my mother, and BFF Liz confirming that attending this retreat was the next step on my journey.

The timing felt perfect as I had just completed an intensive four-day training program in the Grief Recovery Method® and received certification to run groups and do one-on-one sessions. During the program, I worked on and came to completion with my tumultuous relationship with my mother. Seeing signs that pointed me to her assured me we were complete. I was free to love and forgive her.

When the plane landed in Mexico after an extremely long day of travel, I sobbed uncontrollably with profound joy! It felt as if I had returned to my soul's home. I was simultaneously at peace and excited. Although I had never been to this part of Mexico, everything about it felt familiar and comforting, like a well-worn serape. As my driver turned the corner on to the street where my guest house was located, I saw a woman who, from the back, looked exactly like my mother. Another sign from the Universe that I was in the right place.

I sat in the garden courtyard of an old hacienda in San Miguel de Allende. A lovely fountain burbled nearby, its surface filled with hot pink bougainvillea blossoms—so Mexican, so alive! A beautiful gold-colored butterfly landed next to me. It looked like a bronze piece. I bent to touch it, and it started fluttering its wings, startling me. It conjured up the Mexican celebration of the Day of the Dead, which plays homage to deceased ancestors with candies and thousands, maybe millions, of monarch butterflies in the air.

Next to me on the table was a Mexican folk art-looking tissue box with sayings printed on it. They read, "Make this day count,"

167

"Today is a good day to smile," "If you believe it. You can create it," and "I am a limited edition." These messages resonated with me, reminding me to put joy in my life even when I'm grieving. Joy can exist alongside grief. Celebrate life as it is customary to do in Mexico.

Even before the retreat began, I felt grounded and centered, knowing my new path was perfectly aligned. The six-room guesthouse filled with the rest of the wonderful supportive women also seeking. In the program we worked on together, we grew and shared a brilliant experience. We visited art galleries and art installations, bonded over an authentic Mexican cooking experience, laughed, ate, and shared dreams while making vision boards for the next chapter of our life journeys.

This trip to Mexico expanded my solo travel experience; I was more of a risk-taker than ever before, trusted my intuition, was open to the possibilities and the unknown, and learned to give more credence to the intangible in my life. I gained confidence in my command of the Spanish language, finding myself slipping into Spanish often, even in my dreams, and serving as the translator for most of the group and inn staff.

By my last day in San Miguel de Allende, I walked alone into the center of town, stopping to chat with gallery owners and shopkeepers, admiring their wares and finding special gifts to bring home. I even took myself out for a lovely lunch in a small restaurant off the beaten path, feeling totally at home.

These experiences brought me full circle from my first visit to Mexico at age twelve to today as an adult, complete with all the ups and downs, traveling alone as I journey through life. I've grown, I am at peace, and I find joy in experiences, even when they are difficult.

My hope is that you seize the opportunity to find a way to complete your relationships and to bring joy into your life today and every day. I wish you a coming home, coming to completion, and experiencing the same type of joy that I feel daily.

Reflection:

Have you ever visited somewhere that you'd never been before but felt that you had? Describe the feeling and what you learned.

Are you attracted to certain countries, cities, or states? What draws you to them?

How do your ancestors show themselves to you? What messages do they bring?

Remembering My Sacred Self

ANGELA SHAKTI SPARKS

The news that Robin Williams had taken his life came as an utter shock. My heart sank, and intense sadness washed over me. I fondly remembered his movies that had profoundly touched and inspired me. I remembered all of the joy and laughter he brought to the world. How could this happen? Why did this happen?

I've always been sensitive, but this pierced me more deeply than usual. I pictured him alone after all the crowds and friends were gone, sitting with the pain and despair hiding beneath the surface. It resonated deeply because I'd been there.

Memories of my own suffering came flooding back—the years of cyclic depression, intense emotional pain, and seemingly unending traumas and disappointments. Nights alone spent questioning the meaning of life and my purpose (or lack thereof)—years of holding it together on the outside while silently screaming on the inside. I felt like I didn't belong here, and even though I had many friends—as I imagine Robin did too—I felt utterly alone in my pain.

I remembered the night I almost took my life, clutching a bottle of pills in my trembling hands with tears streaming down my face, yearning to escape. When I was in that deep, dark place, I just wanted it to all go away, and, in that moment, death felt like the only way.

In the following years, two friends found themselves in the same place. One was a vivacious performer—full of passion. The other, who attempted but failed, was one of the strongest, most radiant women I knew. She had a successful business and a family.

We all have painful life experiences. I've gone through losing a boyfriend in a car accident, my parents' divorce (which I felt blamed for), verbally abusive relationships, drugs, alcohol, rape, losing my mother, and chronic health conditions since childhood.

I told myself that others had it worse than me. For years, I struggled in silence, feeling unsupported, afraid of being judged, being a burden, or even being worthy of a better life. I incessantly shamed myself for not being able to pull myself out of it.

In the search for love and approval, I compromised my needs, desires, and boundaries in order to please others, submitting to other people's plans, giving in to unwanted sex, and compromising my authenticity.

Over the years, I forgot who I was, the truth of my soul buried deep beneath layers of childhood wounding, indoctrinated beliefs, and societal expectations.

My light was dimmed and my soul heavy under crushing emotions, and my gift of sensitivity as an empath felt like a curse. I did my best to shut it down and numb it out.

Yet, when we shut down, numb, or avoid unpleasant feelings, we are also shutting down our ability to feel love, joy, connection, and all of the uplifting emotions.

To cope, some turn to pharmaceuticals, self-sacrifice to the point of exhaustion, or prove their worth through over-achieving at the cost of their joy and well-being.

Some of us judge, criticize, and self-shame, telling ourselves, "I should have known better, done better, been able to figure it out on my own." Others sink into patterns of emotional eating, drugs, alcohol, excessive shopping, or endless social media scrolling.

Drugs and alcohol were my solace to escape the misery of the world, and I was a master of self-shaming, people-pleasing, avoiding, and isolating. Whatever the maladaptive behaviors are, they keep us stuck, blocking us from the joyful and fulfilling life that is here for us.

This human life comes with loss, disappointment, and situations that shake us to our core. I get how it can tear one down to the point of wanting it all to go away. I intimately understand the overwhelm, exhaustion, despair, and patterns of numbing, avoidance, and distraction.

My pivotal moment came when I found myself once again yearning for death, crying daily and begging the Universe to grant me eternal repose.

One afternoon, after another bout of crying to exhaustion and at the point of possibly losing the few remaining positive aspects of my life, a resolute determination ignited within me. I was finally ready to do whatever it would take to heal my past and liberate myself from the shackles of depression.

Like the heroes and heroines in every inspiring story of transformation, we first look for the easiest path, only to be thwarted at every pass until we accept that the way out is through, as Brené Brown calls it, "the messy middle."

As I dove into the depths of my soul and faced my shadow, I discovered that doing the inner work was way less painful than the struggle, avoidance, and masks I wore. I learned to process emotions, work with my ego rather than fight against it, nurture my wounded inner child, and call back into wholeness the fragmented shards of my soul.

On the other side was glorious freedom. Freedom from physical pain, intense emotional suffering, stories of the past on repeat in my head, and freedom from emotional triggers running my life.

I realized life is a journey of remembrance. Whether suffering from physical afflictions, emotional turmoil, or mental anguish, I believe that at the core, we have forgotten one or more aspects of our truth and are experiencing profound disconnection from it. It stops us from living our authentic, joyful, fulfilling lives.

I was unconsciously disconnected from my emotions, from the harmonious cycles of life, from the divine source within, from my wholeness, and from the essential embrace of connection and community.

I had forgotten my magic and our true essence of love, joy, and oneness.

Fearing judgment, I masked my authentic self, choosing what I thought I should do, ignoring the whispers of my inner guidance and soul's desires.

I criticized and judged myself and my body, conditioned to see myself as less than, and blinded to my body's magnificent innate healing abilities.

Our past actions, emotions, patterns, and conditioned programs and beliefs are not who we are. Yet, these programs, like putting everyone else's wants and needs before our own, run deep. Much of it is so deeply ingrained that it is out of our awareness, which is why I believe it's of utmost importance not to walk the path alone.

Isolating is where it's easiest to fall into an abyss of despair or stay stuck in an uninspired existence. It's the place where we mentally crumble or languish in resentment, anger, or shame. Where some choose to take their life, some come close, and others remain entrenched in their suffering or maladaptive patterns, comfortable in their discomfort.

We can't always see the patterns and beliefs that keep us stuck. While I did much healing work on my own, it was not without the support of guides, coaches, other healers, and holistic health practitioners along the way.

I don't get it right every day, but I give myself grace and remind myself that life ebbs and flows, just as the waves rise and fall and the moon waxes and wanes.

It's a lifelong journey. I continue to develop my practices of living with the cycles and rhythm of life rather than pushing against it. I practice being loving and compassionate with myself instead of judging and criticizing—honoring my wants and needs and maintaining stronger boundaries rather than people-pleasing to the point of exhaustion or resentment. Even as a healer and coach myself, I ask for the support I need instead of self-criticizing for needing it. I stay open to seeing my unconscious patterns so that I may choose differently. I honor my intuition and look for joy in each day.

As I do, life is easier, lighter, and filled with possibilities. More magic and miracles flow in. When I trust in the Universe and my inner guidance, more opportunities arise. Knowing that challenges are catalysts for growth, my past no longer defines me. I stay on the path of growth and evolution with the support of my friends, angels, and guides.

The journey of remembering my sacred self and living my truth has reignited my spirit. As I express my intuitive, adventurous self, a joyous, fulfilling tapestry of life continues to unfold.

May you, dear fellow soul traveler, remember, honor, and live your truth and never walk the path alone.

Reflection:

Have you ever felt disconnected from your feelings?
What did that feel like? What tools did you leverage to
reconnect with yourself?

Describe a situation where you felt stuck. What
happened to get you to that point? How did you get
unstuck?

In what ways have you self-medicated to avoid a
situation? Does this serve you? If not, what might
you try differently?

Editor's Note

DEBORAH KEVIN

Life Shifts. What powerful words. My life has shifted more times than many, partly because of the frequent moves we made during my childhood. I had the opportunity to reinvent myself with each move, but with it came a cost: burying my true self. Fitting in was more important than being authentic. Hiding felt safer.

The problem with hiding was that with each move and reinvention became another layer to push my true nature down. *Deep* down. It wasn't until I had a significant life shift in my forties that I paused to reflect on my role in creating that situation—and decided what I wanted to change to reconnect with my authentic being. Choosing that shift changed the entire trajectory of my life. I went from dwelling in the "muggle" world to living a life of ease, flow, and magic.

The stories in this anthology reflect similar trajectories for the authors in their relationships, with their health, and—most importantly—with themselves. Their courage in sharing their most vulnerable moments and experiences allows our readers to examine their own lives and create their own shifts.

I believe we're at a crossroads. Never before in history has it been more crucial for women to empower themselves and uplift others to do the same. Because we want—no, we *need*—more women to step fully into their power, to light the dark path of uncertainty, and bravely lead where men fear to tread.

For too long, women have stayed in the shadows, working beneath the radar, often staying silent about the things that matter. Now is a time for all women, but in particular, those who have reached midlife, to claim their seats at the table and speak their truths. To share their enlightenment with a troubled world. To spread their love and joy, and freedom. To be queens of their realms.

The women authors in *Life Shifts* share stories of heartbreak, love, discovery, and illness, each trial offering an opportunity for them to transform their experiences, learn from their pain, and grow themselves along the way. May you be drawn to the stories meant to serve, inspire, and uplift you. Use the journal prompts to contemplate, excavate, and shift that in your life which you feel called to.

May these stories bring you to a place of quiet contemplation and then to a place of divine action. The world is waiting for you. The only question before you is: when your life shifts, what magic awaits?

About The Authors

SHA BLACKBURN

Sha Blackburn is an internationally known psychic. She is known to be compassionate, insightful, and "scary accurate." She is passionate about life and helping others to learn, understand, and cope. Sha has been featured on AM, FM, and internet radio since 2003, offering her gifts. She uses her motivation, healing, and psychic abilities to help people transform their lives. Sha was named "Woman of the Year in 2012," by the NAPW, and was named "Inspirational Woman of the Year in 2014" by WRN1 Radio. You can learn more about her at www.LoonWitch.com.

MARIA BURKE

Maria Burke was born in Midleton, County Cork, Ireland. She immigrated to the US in 1988, attended LaBoure College in Milton, and earned her nursing degree. She served as a visiting nurse and soon launched her own home health care company. Celtic Angels has offices in Weymouth and Needham. Her staff, Certified Nursing Assistants, Home Health Aides and Registered Nurses provide a variety of services including skilled nursing, and homemaking services, many other in-home health care services. For more information, please visit www.celticangelsinc.com.

CRYSTAL COCKERHAM

Spiritual mentor, retreat leader, and author, **Crystal Cockerham,** works with empathic women to deepen their relationship with the Divine, learn their souls' language, and hone their empathic gifts so they can create the divinely inspired life they envision, desire, and deserve. Through her offerings and community, Crystal empowers and supports women in awakening their inner wisdom. Learn more at www.CrystalCockerham.com.

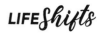

SHARON KATHRYN D'AGOSTINO

Sharon Kathryn D'Agostino is a passionate advocate for the empowerment of women and girls everywhere, and for the human rights of all. She is the founder of the story-sharing platform, SayItForward.org, cohost of *The Power of Stories* podcast with Yodit Kifle Smith, and host of monthly online Women's Circles. Sharon believes in the power of love, compassion, and gratitude, and in our shared responsibility to shape a kinder, gentler, more compassionate world for all. Learn more at www.SayItForward.org.

CAMILLA DE MARIO

Camilla De Mario was born and raised in Milan, Italy. She moved to the United States in 1995. A children's books author, illustrator, artist, screenwriter, and animated films producer, her career evolved from her passion for developing cartoon characters. She lives in Florida, and she is a faculty member of the Vero Beach Museum of Art. She teaches art to children, veterans, and seniors. Learn more at www.CamyDeMario.com.

MARY BETH GUDEWICZ

Intuitive Mary Beth Gudewicz, CNTP, MNT, BCHN, FNLP, CFSP, CGP is the founder of Bella Nutrition Services LLC. As a board-certified functional nutritionist and board-certified holistic nutrition and healthy gut specialist and certified food and spirit practitioner, Mary Beth helps clients get to the root of their health issues—their gut. She compassionately guides clients to soothe their gut and reclaim their optimal health through intuitive guidance, nutritional therapy, and lifestyle shifts. Learn more at www.BellaNutritionServices.com.

LISA HROMADA

Lisa Hromada is an Empowered Lifeview™ guide, Life Transformation mentor, and creator of Love is the Seed™—a spirit-led lifework dedicated to empowering women to harness the power of their minds and align with their souls, so they transcend their challenges and reclaim their joy. Start your journey with her FREE Resources: The Empowered Lifeview™ gift set and Access Your Soul & Life Purpose masterclass at www.LoveIsTheSeed.com.

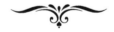

SHERRY KACHANIS

Sherry Kachanis inspires, educates, and empowers others to be their best selves by breaking through unconscious barriers to fully live! She is an experienced energy worker, master neuro linguistics practitioner (NLP), spiritual coach, and mentor with over twenty years of experience guiding and coaching individuals with their spiritual and personal needs. Sherry is also an entrepreneur, public speaker, writer, and artist. Sherry resides in Charleston, SC, with her husband Stewart and their three cats. Learn more at www.SherryKachanis.com.

YVETTE LEFLORE

Yvette LeFlore is an intuitive energy healer, Reiki master teacher, and crystal clinician. Yvette's mission is to support people to fill their energetic cups to overflowing so they have enough to give others without depleting themselves. She particularly enjoys working with folks who are on the "front line" (social justice, parents, teachers, nurses, etc.) because they so often have depleted themselves for the sake of their jobs or passions. She offers group and individualized healings. Yvette lives in Salem, Virginia, with her husband and two four-legged healing partners, Jasper and Cleo. Learn more at www.HealingWithYvette.com.

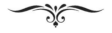

MICHELLE LEMOI

Transformational and evolutionary guide **Michelle Lemoi** is passionately dedicated to supporting women in reconnecting with their feminine essence, getting off autopilot, and releasing pushing, doing, and striving tendencies. Her deepest desire is that women discover that within them is the ability to create success, balance, and more joy in their lives from a place of authenticity, truth, and inner peace. As a visionary leader, speaker, media guest, and bestselling contributing author, Michelle provides workshops, programs, and events for women ready to say "Yes" to embracing their inner power and "No" to the constraints in their lives. www.MichelleLemoi.com.

AMY LINDNER-LESSER

Grief Recovery Method® specialist and certified life transitions coach **Amy Lindner-Lesser, MSW,** compassionately supports women through the emotions of loss and grief that arise with major life transitions. Whether it's the heartbreaking grief that arises from the loss of a loved one or the disorientation felt when life suddenly shifts due to the loss of a job, relationship, identity, or a health challenge, Amy is passionate about guiding clients to understand and navigate the transition with self-compassion. Learn more at www.INNtrospection.com.

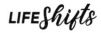

MARY MAGOUIRK

Conscious Choices coach **Mary Magouirk** empowers and teaches her clients how to make conscious choices that align their thoughts, beliefs, and actions with the dreams and vision they hold for their life. As a master law of attraction coach and desire factor coach, Mary's unique methodology, empowering use of storytelling, and her supportive non-judgmental coaching style supports clients in understanding where their predominant vibration is and how they can consciously choose to create the outcomes that they desire. Learn more at www.LifeJustBeyond.com.

KAREN MCPHAIL

Karen McPhail is a soulmate manifestation coach, certified life coach, certified Infinite Possibilities trainer with Mike Dooley, certified quantum manifestation coach and creator of the highly successful twelve-week women's program, *The Soulmate Solution*, where she empowers women to manifest their soulmate partner while becoming their own soulmate and loving their lives in the process. As a life coach, she supports individuals to clearly define, create, and achieve their dream lives. Learn more at www.InfiniteLifePossibilities.com.

CYNTHIA MEDINA

A certified transformational life and health coach and energy practitioner, **Cynthia Medina** has been dedicated to the emotional, spiritual, and physical well-being of women for over twenty years. She intuitively combines her knowledge and training in Ayurveda, naturopathy, meditation, NLP, Reiki, hypnosis, and other modalities to support women in breaking through the emotional and energetic blocks to healing and success. Cynthia works with clients individually and in her group programs. Learn more at www.CoachCynthiaMedina.com.

FELICIA MESSINA-D'HAITI

Felicia Messina-D'Haiti is a feng shui practitioner and certified soul coach, whose passion is to support people in clearing the physical, mental, emotional and spiritual blockages that hinder them from living a life of freedom, balance, joy and to where their soul leads. Felicia is an award-winning educator, Interior Alignment® Feng Shui and Space Clearing Master Teacher and Soul Coaching® Trainer. She is an *Aspire Magazine* Expert Columnist and contributing author to several bestselling books. Learn more at www.FeliciaDHaiti.com.

NANCY OKEEFE

Nancy OKeefe is a certified quantum human design specialist, intuitive business coach, and compassionate transformer, who helps women entrepreneurs peel back the layers of who they have been taught to be and how they have been conditioned to do business so they can live their inner truth and build an abundant and sustainable business that feeds their soul. Learn more at www. NancyOKeefeCoaching.com.

MARY JO RATHGEB

Mary Jo Rathgeb, life transitions coach and certified RIM facilitator, helps clients shine a light on shadow emotions so they can reclaim the energy and wisdom within. Mary Jo holds space for, and expertly guides, women who are ready to release people-pleasing and perfectionism so they can align their lives with their authentic selves. She specializes in working with women catalyzed by major life changes who want to navigate it consciously. Learn more at www.MaryJoRathgeb.com.

KAREN SHIER

Karen Shier is a midlife transformation guide, Desire Factor and Law of Attraction life coach, energy master, and author who guides women in releasing what no longer lights them up, so they can joyfully thrive in the second halves of their lives. She is passionate about supporting women in moving from feeling stuck, stressed, and unhappy to feeling free, empowered, and ready to co-create a marvelous life. Learn more at www.KarenShierCoaching.com.

BONNIE SNYDER

Merging thirty-years of psychology and energy-based trainings, Intuitive Life Balance coach and Energy Psychology Diplomat Bonnie Snyder, Ed.S., CPC, DCEP, supports overwhelmed highly sensitive women to uncover and release their limiting thoughts and beliefs so they can embrace their sensitivities as the superpowers that they are. She compassionately meets her clients where they are and intuitively chooses from her many modalities, such as self-havening, Donna Eden energy medicine, positive psychology and EFT to name a few. Learn more at www.DiamondPathways.com

ANGELA SHAKTI SPARKS

Angela Shakti Sparks is an intuitive channel, energy healer, EFT tapping, NLP practitioner, and yoga instructor, who is devoted to empowering women to thrive with renewed energy and purpose. She supports female entrepreneurs in transcending stress, overwhelm, physical and mental exhaustion, and the pressure of managing multiple roles and responsibilities. By revitalizing their energy and guiding them in cultivating a more harmonious work-life balance, fempreneurs realign with their innate creativity, flow, health, passion, and joy. Learn more at www.AngelaShaktiSparks.com.

ROSA MARIA SZYNSKI

Rosa Maria Szynski is a Magical Living Mentor™ and Creative Dream Guide™. Through storytelling and intuitive wisdom, she invites women to tune in to their own heart and wake up to their dreams. Her transformational M.A.G.I.C.A.L process leads women on a journey of self-discovery to awaken the beauty, love, and magic within. Rosa is the author of *Love Letters: An Inspirational Guide to Sending Messages of Love, Changing the Way We Communicate.* Learn more at www.RadiancewithRosa.com.

CINDY WINSEL

Cindy Winsel is an artist, teacher, and creative depth life coach. She collaborates with women using powerful tools and approaches and offers her clients ways to engage in their journey. Women in a transitional period in their lives who are looking for a different path to discover their greatest gifts are guided and coached on their journey using expressive arts, SoulCollage,® JourneyCircles,® and other modalities that are the best fit. Learn more at www.CindyWinsel.com.

LEE MURPHY WOLF

Lee Murphy Wolf is the creator of The Calibrate Method,™ which helps soul-led women to define their next chapter in life and business. She shows her clients how to unlock the power of tuning to reconnect with themselves, so they can tap into their wisdom, confidently make aligned choices, and expand. Learn more about her services at www.LeeMurphyWolf.com.

About Our Publisher

LINDA JOY

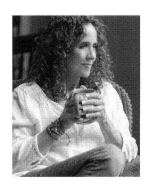

Founded in 2010 by Sacred Visibility™ Catalyst, Mindset Elevation Coach, and *Aspire Magazine* publisher Linda Joy, Inspired Living Publishing, LLC (ILP), is a best-selling boutique hybrid publishing company.

Dedicated to publishing books for women and by women and to spreading a message of love, positivity, feminine wisdom, and self-empowerment to women of all ages, backgrounds, and life paths—ILPs books have reached numerous international bestsellers lists as well as Amazon's Movers & Shakers lists.

The company's authors benefit from Linda's family of multimedia inspirational brands that reach over 44,000 subscribers and social media community.

ILP works with mission-driven, heart-centered female entrepreneurs—life, business, and spiritual coaches, therapists, service providers, and health practitioners in the personal and spiritual development genres, to bring their message and mission to life and to the world.

193

Through ILPs highly successful sacred anthology division, hundreds of visionary female entrepreneurs have written their sacred soul stories using ILP's Authentic Storytelling™ writing model and become bestselling authors.

What sets Inspired Living Publishing™™™ apart is its powerful, high-visibility publishing, marketing, bestseller launch, and exposure across multiple media platforms included in its publishing packages. Their family of authors reap the benefits of being a part of a sacred family of inspirational multimedia brands that deliver the best in transformational and empowering content across a wide range of platforms—and has been doing so since 2006 with the birth of *Aspire Magazine.*

Linda also works privately with empowered female entrepreneurs and messengers through her Illuminate Sistermind™ Program and other visibility-enhancing offerings. Linda's other inspirational brands include Inspired Living Secrets,™ Inspired Living Giveaway,™ and her popular radio show, Inspired Conversations. Learn more about Linda's private work and offerings at www.Linda-Joy.com.

Learn how you can be a part of one of our sacred anthologies at **www.InspiredLivingPublishing.com.**

About Our Editor

DEBORAH KEVIN

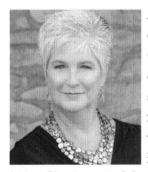 As the founder and chief inspiration officer of Highlander Press, Deborah Kevin (pronounced "KEY-vin") loves helping change-makers tap into and share their stories of healing and truth with impactful books. She's trekked over 350 miles of the Camino de Santiago and her passions include travel, cooking, hiking, and kayaking. She lives in Maryland with the love of her life, Rob, their sons, and their puppy Fergus—that is when they're not off discovering the world. Learn more at www.DeborahKevin.com.

ABOUT THE EDITOR

About Our Editor

ADAM S. KAROFSKY

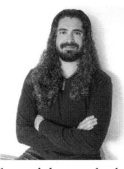

Adam S. Karofsky is a writer, editor, and business owner of his company, ASK Writes. A lifelong lover of stories and mythology, Adam helps others tell their tales by ghostwriting, rewriting, and editing the written word. After studying anthropology at the University of Massachusetts Amherst's Commonwealth Honors College, Adam embarked on several multi-month trips around the world, including Central America, Europe, the Middle East, and the United States.

Made in the USA
Columbia, SC
05 November 2023

25306073R00120